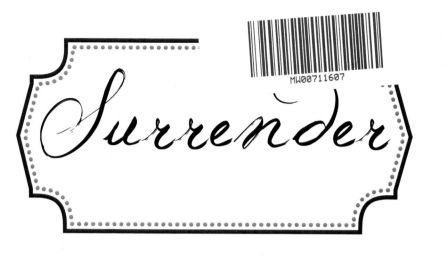

Surrender

To: Rebas

Praying you well

be encouraged by

what God has done!

Amy Hanley

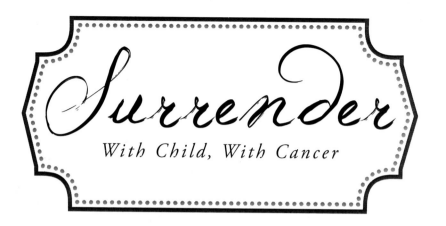

Surrender

With Child, With Cancer

AMY HANLEY

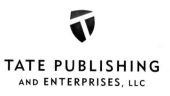

TATE PUBLISHING
AND ENTERPRISES, LLC

Published by Tate Publishing & Enterprises, LLC
127 E. Trade Center Terrace | Mustang, Oklahoma 73064 USA
1.888.361.9473 | www.tatepublishing.com

Tate Publishing is committed to excellence in the publishing industry. The company reflects the philosophy established by the founders, based on Psalm 68:11,
"The Lord gave the word and great was the company of those who published it."

Book design copyright © 2013 by Tate Publishing, LLC. All rights reserved.
Cover design by Rhezette Fiel
Interior design by Jomar Ouano

Published in the United States of America

ISBN: 978-1-62746-218-1
1. Medical / Diseases / Cancer See Oncology
2. Religion / Christian Life / Inspirational
13.05.28

Acknowledgments

I would first and foremost like to thank my God, my Lord and Savior, Jesus Christ, for choosing me, touching me, and healing me. My prayer is that my life will always bring glory to you.

To Bobby, Jonathan, Luke, Emma, and Joshua, I love you more than words can say. Thank you for your love, support, encouragement, understanding, and patience.

To my mom, extended family, and our many dear friends, there are no words sufficient enough to describe my gratitude for all you have done.

Thank you to my very dear oncologist for taking a chance on me. You will forever hold a special place in our hearts.

Disclaimer

Names have been changed to protect the privacy of individuals who may wish to remain anonymous.

The decisions that I made were based on personal and religious beliefs. I am not a physician and am in no way suggesting that a person should disregard the advice of medical professionals.

Contents

Foreword

In the fall of 2009, I was living the life of which dreams are made. I had the privilege of being at home with my children, educating them, training them, and just spending time with them. I had married the man that God had made for me, to complement my personality and make me complete.

I met Bobby in the spring of 1996. It was a set up, a blind date arranged by one of his cousins. He was a good ole boy reminding me of the Hank Williams Jr. song "A Country Boy Can Survive." This city girl knew it must be love when after dating for only a few short months, Bobby invited me along for a rabbit hunting expedition. I was impressed with his accuracy with his rifle until after much success, he inquired, "Can you hold his feet while I skin him?" Too shocked to speak and not wanting him to see my horror and disgust, I slowly nodded my head. Eating rabbit mull for supper, this urbanite knew I was either crazy or in love. Maybe it was just crazy in love!

Bobby is the easygoing type. I, on the other hand, have a tendency to become hysterical with very little cause. He is the problem solver while I am frequently the problem causer with my strong, high-strung personality. He keeps me levelheaded, and I encourage him. We have a traditional, old-fashioned marriage, where he is the provider and I am the keeper of our home. Having come from a broken home, I had dreamed of having a family of my own. This was my dream in real life. We weren't rich, but we had all we needed, and we were happy.

Fulfillment comes in different forms for different people. For me, fulfillment is simply defined as being a wife and mom. I am fulfilled every day that I spend as Bobby's wife and being mom to Jonathan, eleven; Luke, seven; Emma, five; and Joshua, ten months. Before becoming a mom, I loved my job as a schoolteacher.

When Bobby and I married, he was working as a civil engineer for local county government. I was teaching middle school. We had things planned so perfectly. Our careers were on the fast track. In five years' time, we could own our home and be living debt-free; then it would be the perfect time to start a family. Well, God had another plan for us. Just a little over a year after the beginning of our perfect plan, God gave us Jonathan. I had planned to continue my job as an educator, but all those plans suddenly changed with a small cry, a soft touch, and a sweet smell. The first time I held Jonathan, I knew that I wasn't going back to the classroom anytime soon. Financially, resigning from my job was the worst decision that we ever made. For our family, it was the best. With Bobby's consent, I turned in my resignation and embarked on the most rewarding job on earth.

Being a mom has been the greatest joy that I have ever known. Jonathan (gracious gift of God) has been a delight in so many ways. He is a tall, skinny, dirty-blond headed, blue-eyed version of me. The boy couldn't sit still if his life depended on it. He loves to be outside. Because we home-school him, he gets to spend more time in the outdoors than most kids. He does as little academically as he feels he can get away with and then he runs for the door, not to return until thirst and hunger overtake him or it gets dark, whichever comes first. There is an unending trail of building projects and invention in the backyard, reflecting his creativity and work ethic. Jonathan has the most compassionate, loving heart, always concerning himself with the needs of others. He is responsible and trustworthy, just the type of young man to make any mother proud.

When Jonathan was four, our family grew again as we added a blue-eyed, red-haired bundle of joy named Luke (giver of light). Luke has more of his dad's temperament. What a relief! He is laid-back, never getting particularly worked up over small stuff. Luke is less of a talker and more of a thinker. The problem solver, he reasonably draws conclusions by rationalizing. As my studious child, his love for learning makes being his teacher easy. Luke loves gardening and looks forward to starting our garden each spring. After the plowing and planting are completed, he anxiously awaits for the first plants to pop up. He monitors, waters, and pulls weeds around the tender young plants. Watching and waiting for the first of the harvest, he checks daily for blooms and fruit. Luke is a hard worker, giving his all in everything he does, whether it is playing baseball, growing a garden, or his academics. Always willing to help when needed and a pleasant company to keep, Luke is a blessing to our family.

Two years after Luke was born, Emma (industrious) made her arrival. With two boys, we were delighted that God had given us a girl this time. Emma is a loving young lady, full of personality! She enjoys helping to take care of others. She helps Jonathan keep up with his things, ties Luke's shoes for him, and brings Daddy a cold glass of water when he is working outside. At five years old, Emma makes biscuits and tea and is always ready to help with supper. She truly is a well-rounded girl. She can be very prissy in her fancy clothes and hair bows tied neatly in her long, blond hair, but she also likes her cammo jeans, can bait her own hook, hits a baseball as well as most boys, and is the first one up and dressed to go hunting in the fall. She is tough when she plays, but tender in her heart. Emma keeps us all on our toes with her high energy level and assertiveness. There is never a dull moment where there lives a ray of sunshine named Emma.

With Emma's arrival, our family was complete (or so we thought). Things were good. Bobby's career was a great success both professionally and financially. I was happy at home supporting Bobby in his career and raising the children.

What was to come would be life changing in ways that we never could have fathomed. Only God knew from before the beginning to the end the what, why, how, and when of our looming sickness. All we knew was the Who.

Omniscience

God began preparing me for the coming storm months before it began. The experiences that God puts in our paths are often preparation for a greater purpose to be revealed in his time. In November 2009, the storm clouds began to gather when I suffered another miscarriage. It was my second. The questions encircled me as grief began to swallow me. Why did God take my baby again? I was a good mother. I wanted this baby. Why did this happen to me? It seemed almost cruel for God to allow me to become pregnant again just to snatch away the precious life that was growing inside of me.

It took only a taste of the evening news to make me angry. With bitterness building inside of me, I watched story after story of neglect and child abuse. I became angry with God. One mother, it was reported, had left her newborn baby in a public toilet to die. Yet God had taken *my* baby. Furious, I screamed over and over to God, "This is not fair!" I had yet to understand that God saw a bigger picture, one to which I was not privy.

I did not understand that God was teaching me, preparing me. First, God was reiterating the sanctity of human life, showing me that all life is created by him and for his purpose. Secondly, in the midst of my grief and despair, God was showing me that he has a plan for everything. My suffering occurred for a reason, and God knew what he was doing. It turned out that the baby that I lost ultimately saved my life.

It was during this pregnancy that I began to have some suspicious health symptoms. A small amount of bleeding began to show up with bowel movements. Hemorrhoids are not uncommon in pregnancy, so I assumed they were the culprit. I was not alarmed. Young and active, I led a healthy lifestyle and felt good. With three young children to care for, I did not have the time nor the inclination to worry. I decided that if the bleeding continued after I gave birth, then I would consider going to the doctor.

I never gave birth. I lost the baby at eight weeks when a routine ultrasound revealed that the baby I was carrying was not growing and there was no heartbeat. As my body was beginning to heal from the trauma of the miscarriage, the bleeding from my rectum continued. With growing concern, my husband then insisted that I needed to be checked by a doctor. So at his urging and the urging of other friends, I made the appointment.

Still grieving from the miscarriage that I had just experienced, I prayed daily for another baby. God called me instead to a place of surrender. If it was his will for me to have another baby, then I would. If not, then it was his will for me to rest in contentment with what he had given to me and to live in peace desiring only his will. It is so hard sometimes to surrender to God something that we want so badly. I began to pray for God to align my wants up with his will.

Once I surrendered my right to have another baby—I'm talking truly giving up my dream—God spoke to me. It was on a Sunday morning while we were getting ready for church. I had begged God for another child, but after he had dealt with my heart, I had relinquished my dream. Funny how it often seems it is merely our willingness to die to self for his purpose that God requires. So God spoke to me. I don't know exactly how to describe it. For those who have had this type of experience, it is easy to understand. A knowing of sorts came over me in an overwhelming sense of the presence of God. I knew in that moment that I was pregnant; it was a boy, and his name was to be Joshua. I went straight to Bobby sharing this revelation with my husband as he sat quietly with the deepest look of concern on his face.

He was sitting at the kitchen table eating a bowl of cereal. I began hesitantly, searching for the right words so that I would not scare him. I had only gotten out the part about being pregnant when he began to choke. Once he had dislodged the cocoa puff, he asked me if I happened to recall just how old we were. When I explained that I had no scientific evidence to support my pregnancy claim, he relaxed. His concern then shifted to the state of my sanity.

Realizing his concern, I simply suggested that he wait and see. I knew beyond the shadow of any doubt that God had spoken. Several weeks later, my pregnancy was confirmed. I could not resist at least one small "I told you so." My baby was a boy, and his name had to be Joshua, meaning "God saves." However, at the time I could not understand the significance of the name.

Sickness

It took several weeks to get an appointment to see a doctor. While waiting, our concern grew as the bleeding that I had been experiencing continued. At the first visit I had with Dr. Kay, a gastroenterologist, she listened intently as I explained my symptoms. She felt very strongly that I had a condition called colitis. In fact, she was 85 percent sure. We would go ahead, however, and schedule a sigmoidoscopy, a procedure in which a device is used to view the inside walls of the colon, in an attempt to confirm her preliminary diagnosis. I went home that day and researched colitis online. It was not something I was excited about having, but most cases appeared to be controllable by diet. I needed to be on a better diet anyway, I thought.

I was six weeks pregnant with Joshua when I went for the sigmoidoscopy. Because of my pregnancy, no anesthesia was used. Therefore, I was fully awake and aware as the procedure began. It was uncomfortable, but bearable. I watched the procedure on the screen along with the doctor and the nurses. Nothing extraordinary appeared as I heard my doctor comment that she wasn't seeing what she had expected. She then told me that this did not look like colitis. I asked her, "If it isn't colitis, then what is causing the bleeding?" She answered me, "I don't know yet, I am still looking." She continued the examination. Then I saw it at the same time she did. A bloody mass was on the wall of my colon. The tissue was soft, she explained, not likely to be cancer. She would do a biopsy just to be sure. Dr. Kay told me and my husband that she was 98 percent sure this was not cancer. "Go home and don't worry," she advised. We were to expect the results of the biopsy in about a week.

Exactly four days later, I had just arrived home from taking Emma, my daughter, to dance class, when I hit Play on the answering machine and heard the message that would ultimately turn my world upside down. It was the voice of Dr. Kay's receptionist telling me to be in her office the next morning and to bring my husband. I suddenly felt lightheaded, knowing that this could not be good. Trying to comfort myself, I reasoned that the doctor was 98 percent sure that I did not have cancer. This receptionist must not realize how frightening her message sounded. I considered that perhaps I should speak to my doctor about how her office staff had scared me half to death.

Just to be on the safe side though, I called my husband and some dear Christian friends to request prayer support. Bobby came home from work immediately. As soon as he walked in the door, I felt myself begin to relax. In an effort to comfort me, he agreed that it was probably nothing. That evening, we decided that we would meet with our close friends at a local McDonald's to spend some time together in prayer. Our families enjoyed chocolate and caramel sundaes and a time of fellowship and prayer for my health.

The night that ensued was long with nervousness and sleeplessness. I battled with reason. It was most likely nothing. The thought that it could be something, however, just would not leave me alone. Cancer? It couldn't be. I was too young. This type of thing wouldn't really happen to me, would it? I had heard about things like this occasionally happening to other people, but not to someone I actually knew.

From the time Jonathan was a baby, it had always been my prayer that God would let me live to see my children grow into adulthood. One of my biggest fears had always been of dying while my children were young and still needed me. Only the year before, there was a little boy of about five years old on Luke's baseball team whose mother had passed away suddenly, leaving behind three young children, that she, like me, had been home-schooling. Our family prayed for that family every night for over a year. I pitied the children and the dad. Thinking of them often, I wondered if there was anything I could do to help them. I really never had known them personally. So the only thing that I knew to do was to pray for them. Pray for them, we did.

Eventually, morning came. We arrived at the doctor's office promptly at 9:00 a.m. and were quickly whisked into a room to await the arrival of Dr. Kay. My husband excused himself to the restroom, and of course, the doctor came in while he was out. Being a no-nonsense type of woman, she quietly and quickly took the seat across from me, and getting straight to the point, she looked me in the eye and announced, "You have cancer!" Her tone of voice reflected her own shock as my face surely reflected mine. Bobby, upon returning to the room, quietly closed the door and looked at me with the question clearly reflected in his eyes; he waited. His eyes searched mine, and without a word, he knew. I nodded in confirmation of his worst fear.

Cancer? She had been so sure that it was not cancer. I was so young. Only thirty-eight years old with colon cancer? How could this be? Wasn't colon cancer an older-person disease? Doctors don't even start to screen for colon cancer until fifty years old. Yet my doctor sat here explaining to me that this cancer had been growing in my body for years. I'd had no symptoms. No clues existed to indicate that my body was betraying me. I later learned that the most common symptom of colon cancer is no symptom at all! My doctor told me that my children would need to start screening for colon cancer at twenty-eight years old. There is supposedly a genetic factor involved. This was confusing to me as no one on either side of my family had ever been diagnosed with cancer.

What about how my friends and family had prayed the night before? Didn't God hear those prayers? Why was he allowing this to happen to me? Yet here I was, pregnant.

Pregnant and with cancer. It was decided by my doctor that the best course of action would be for me to have surgery the following week to remove the affected section of my colon. In the meantime, I was to have more testing in preparation for surgery. An MRI was scheduled in an attempt to determine if the cancer had already spread to areas outside of my colon. I arrived at the hospital feeling very uptight. I suffer from a touch of claustrophobia and had heard horror stories about the enclosure that I would be required to lie in for the MRI. Being fearful of what might be found, I was sick with nervousness. Upon checking in, I sat wringing my hands as we waited for the nurse to call my name. Once called, I undressed and donned a hospital gown to be worn for the MRI. Carefully tying the back so as not to flash anyone in the hall, I waited for the nurse to return to retrieve me. When she returned, I was escorted to the testing room where I climbed up on the table to assume the position that I would remain in for the hour-long test. The MRI would first be performed without the contrast that was to be administered through the IV, giving the doctor a clearer look at my abdomen. If needed, the test would be repeated with the contrast. The technician carefully explained to me the importance of lying perfectly still. Once in position, she began to slide me into the machine. I panicked. Only a few feet in, I demanded to be slid back out. We tried again. Same result. This was not going so well. I asked the technician if Bobby could be allowed to come into the room to offer me comfort.

He was the only hope I had of calming me to a point that I would be able to finish the test. Realizing the importance of my completing the MRI, Bobby came through for me. He stood behind the MRI machine as I put my arms up over my head and through the tube reaching out to him. As I began again to slide into the donut hole, I kept my eyes on him with my hands reaching until finally I could reach him. He took my hands, reassuring me, as the test began.

Coming to life, the machine moaned and groaned loudly. Bobby began to dance for me to the rhythmic creaking and banging of the machine. I laughed, trying hard to be still. The hour-long test passed quickly as my husband continued to entertain me. Once completed, the nurse told me that the test would not need to be repeated with contrast. I figured that to be good. On one hand, it means that no cancer was found outside of my colon; therefore the doctor didn't need a closer look. On the other hand, if I was already eaten up with cancer, the doctor might not need a closer look. Waiting for the results was physically and emotionally painful. The results were due back on a Friday. I began calling the doctor's office first thing in the morning, but the doctor was not in the office this particular morning, and the nurse wasn't allowed to discuss the test results with me until after she had spoken to the doctor. As the day wore on, I became fearful that I would be left to face an entire weekend wondering what the MRI had revealed. Crying, I called the nurse yet again, begging her not to make me suffer all weekend. I could not stand the unknown. I desperately needed answers. She worked late that Friday for me to give me the answers that I sought. At 5:30 p.m., when I believed all hope was gone, she returned my call to tell me that the MRI looked great, showing no additional cancer.

Next, I had a full colonoscopy. Preparing for a colonoscopy when pregnant is tough, especially during the first trimester when morning sickness is still so prevalent! In preparation, I was required to drink the "prep" that would clean out my colon, making it possible for my doctor to get a clear look at the colon wall. Every swallow of the prep fought to come back up. I lost that battle many times. Afraid that I wasn't keeping enough down to completely clean me out, we prayed. My friend, Donna, stayed on the phone with me for half of the night praying that prep down. I swallow and gagged, she prayed. It was only by her prayers that I was successful in drinking the sludge. Weak and sick, I made it to the hospital the next morning. The colonoscopy could not have gone better. With neither the MRI nor the colonoscopy revealing any additional areas for concern, my surgery was scheduled.

During the week between my diagnosis and my surgery, I was crippled with fear. Trying to stay busy in an effort of distraction, I cleaned out closets, drawers, the filing cabinet, and I cooked, a lot! I spent time playing with my children and enjoying them as I tried to prepare for the coming separation from them. The nights I spent on my knees asking God to speak to me through his Word. I never sat down with the Bible intentionally searching for arbitrary healing verses. If a healing verse was given to me, it would be from God. Instead, I continued my daily devotions as I had been studying before my diagnosis. The morning after I had received my diagnosis, I was reading in Psalms. Psalms is my favorite book in the Bible. I love the picture it gives us of David's human nature, God's forgiveness and restoration, and God's faithfulness. I had been reading through the Psalms (NIV) and found myself in chapter 30. Verse 2 of chapter 30 says, "Oh, Lord, my God, I cried out to you for help and You healed me." Wow! I believed then as I do now, that God was speaking to me. My confidence grew that I was going to be healed. So confident was I, in fact, that I wrote Psalms 30:2 on the palm of my hand on the morning of my surgery. I wanted to be a witness for God. I wanted the nurses and doctors in the operating room to see that I knew my healing came from the Lord.

Surgery

When I arrived at the hospital for surgery, I was seven weeks pregnant. Terrified, I clung to God with praise. I sang in my heart praises to my Lord. God was with me. His presence surrounded me, giving me a peace that passes all possible understanding. The fear that weighed on me was not that cancer would remain in my body after surgery but rather of losing the baby that I was carrying. I was also extremely anxious about being away from my three children whom I had to leave at home. Because we home-school, my children had never been separated from me. An hour here or there for an appointment or special occasion was the only time I had ever left them. Now we were talking about days. I had to make myself think about something else. No matter how badly I hated to leave them, there was nothing I could do about it. I had to have this surgery.

To be separated from my children was going to be stressful for me and them. The surgeon had told me that I should expect to stay in the hospital for three to five days. Not sure that I could stand to be away from my family for that long, I decided that I would go home in two days! I have always had a certain determination about me, and I had no intention of taking three to five days to get back to my life. Clinging to my verse, I was certain that I would come out of the operating room cancer-free. The last thing I said to my husband was "I will see you on the other side of this cancer thing." I was anxious to get home and continue my life, to prepare for another baby, and to enjoy the family life that Bobby and I had created.

After one last kiss and an "I love you" from my husband, I was wheeled away. Dr. Calvin, my surgeon, attempted to do the entire procedure using laparoscopy. Unfortunately, that was not possible because there was a baby in the way. The surgery was slow, but Dr. Calvin successfully removed a section of my colon measuring about 8 cm. He was also able to complete a resection at the time of the surgery, sparing me the further trauma of having to adjust to wearing an ostomy bag. I suppose it would be accurate to say that the surgery was successful. Immediately following, Dr. Calvin expressed to Bobby that the surgery "went well" and that he believed he had "gotten it all."

The first memory that I have following surgery is of the nurses scurrying around me. I vaguely recall opening my eyes briefly as I heard one of the nurses exclaim, "There it is!" I listened, hearing a quick, faint thumping. I knew immediately what I was hearing. At only seven weeks pregnant, I could hear the tiny pitter patter of a little bitty heart already beating.

I laid there listening as tears of happiness and relief rolled down my face. I began to praise God for his protection over this precious baby. Relief washed over me as joy filled my soul with the knowledge that my baby had survived! I closed my eyes and drifted back to ignorant bliss. The next time I awoke, I was in a private room and as sick as I have ever been in my entire life!

I had been given morphine for pain. The room was spinning. Every time I tried to open my eyes, I began to throw up. Hours passed before I realized that the morphine could be the cause of my sickness and dizziness. At about 2:00 a.m., I requested that the morphine be stopped. The nurse advised against stopping it as she explained to me that she would have no authority to give me anything else for pain until the doctor arrived in the morning. At my insistence, the morphine drip was finally disabled. It was eight hours later when I got my next dose of pain medication. I was hurting, but at least the room had stopped spinning.

As my mind began to clear, my husband excitedly told me how the surgeon had indicated that he believed he had gotten it all. I was not particularly impressed because I had expected as much. God had told me that he was going to heal me in Psalms 30:2, and I believed him. I began fighting to get well so that I could return home and resume my life. My baby had survived the surgery; I was filled with joy. The cancer, I thought, was gone. It was time to move forward. I did not have time to be sick. I had children waiting at home for Mom.

Just a couple of days following the surgery, Dr. Kay came for a visit. How nice of her, I'd thought, as she declared that this was a personal visit. Assuming that we had been given the pathology results, she wanted to check on me. It did not take her long to ascertain that we had not been given the results. She asked us directly, "Has anyone discussed the pathology report with you?" I told her no, we were not expecting the results for a few more days. Realizing that she was now going to be the one to deliver the news, her demeanor changed as she pulled up a chair. She frankly stated, "Well, I have seen it, and it is not good." *What?* I will never forget those words. I have heard them played over and over in my head more times than I can count. I began to feel that familiar nauseated feeling again. She continued, explaining that the cancer had spread, I had a positive lymph node. After consulting with other doctors, she assured me that abortion was my only option. I had to kill my baby and fight for my life. As the room began again to spin, I fought back the overwhelming urge to vomit.

I looked across the room and saw my husband standing in the corner, leaning against the wall, weeping. Oh my goodness, I thought, seeing him sobbing was all the confirmation that I needed that I was about to die. This man, whom I had been with for fourteen years, was crying. In fourteen years I had only seen him cry once. I knew he did not cry easily. I looked at him in stunned amazement. Although I was having trouble following the conversation that he was having with the doctor, I had no trouble sizing up the seriousness of a situation that would cause *this* man to cry with racking sobs.

Initially, Bobby was told that I had a 45 percent chance for survival if I terminated my pregnancy and began treatments immediately. At that time, we were given no hope for survival if I decided to have my baby. The ob-gyn that I was seeing, Dr. Wolf, along with Dr. Kay, explained to us that my pregnancy would cause my cancer to be more aggressive. Delaying treatment, even for the duration of the pregnancy, was not an option if I wanted to survive. On the other hand, my immune system would be compromised by my pregnancy and therefore would not be able to tolerate treatment. I was told that if I attempted treatment during the pregnancy, the baby and I would both die. Dr. Wolf even went so far as to tell me that it would be a slow and painful death for me and the baby. We were left with only one option if I wanted to survive: to kill my baby.

Where was God? How could I have so completely misunderstood him? I thought he had promised me healing. Where did I go wrong? How could God let this happen to me? I lived for him. I had been obedient to his Word and trusted him in our decision for me to give up a rewarding career to be a stay-at-home mom. I home-schooled my children and tried to honor him through their education. How could God do this to my husband? To my children? Where was God? Although I could not answer these questions at that time, there were two things of which I was sure. First, I knew that God had created this life that was growing inside of me, and he had a purpose for this baby. I did not create this baby, God did. It was his child, not mine. How could I even consider killing God's baby? Secondly, I was sure that God knew that I had cancer before I got pregnant. This situation came as no surprise to him. I was certain that God had the power to save me and the baby if that was his will. The problem was that I was no longer sure that it was his will to heal me. Regardless of the apparent hopelessness of the present situation I had found myself in, I still knew that God was in control.

As far as I was concerned, there was no decision to make. I had a baby, not a choice. I would not stand before a holy God one day and have to affirm that, "Yes, Lord, I killed your baby because I didn't trust you." I was having a baby and trusting that God would spare my life. If he did not spare my life—well, I could not let myself consider that possibility yet. I only had enough strength to survive in the moment.

To say that I was sick would be the understatement of the century. Funny thing about the surgical ward at the hospital, they have no idea what to do with a pregnant woman. Being that I was in my first trimester, I was suffering from a pretty substantial case of morning sickness. Add medication and a liquid diet to morning sickness, and you have one sick mama! The hospital would not let me have solid food until I stopped throwing up. However, I could not stop until I got something in my pregnant stomach to settle it. It was an unfortunate cycle that left me sick and weak. Not seeing any hope for the situation to change and with me begging him, Bobby sneaked in a pack of soda crackers for me to eat. That did the trick. I stopped throwing up. It was decided that I could have my first real meal following surgery. It was breakfast. The hospital cafeteria staff delivered my breakfast plate. I have never been so hungry in my entire life! My mouth watered as I prepared to take the lid off of my plate and reveal what deliciousness was being offered to me. Oh, the horror as I uncovered southwestern scrambled eggs! One whiff and back to the trash can I went. Immediately, the nurse took my tray and declared that I was obviously still not ready for solid food. So the cycle continued.

Day after day went by without me being able to see my children. I had been too sick for them to see me in the beginning. Days ran together as I drifted in and out of consciousness, not realizing how long I had been in the hospital. Unaware of what was going on in the world outside of my hospital room, I didn't even know that it had snowed. Living in Georgia all my life, it is rare that we get enough snow to really play in, and I had missed it. My cousin Anna took photos of my children playing in the snow and brought them to me at the hospital. I treasured those pictures dearly.

I had many visitors, family, and friends who came to support us. These dear friends prayed with us and offered any help that could be given in a situation like ours. One particular incidence stood out above the rest. My uncle and aunt along with some cousins came to visit. They, like us, had felt shell-shocked at my prognosis. Discussion began about an attempt to get me to MD Anderson, one of the world's leading cancer centers. If there was any hope for me, this certainly would be the best source. But money has never come to us in abundance. We have always had everything that we needed, but we lived pay check to pay check like many other families. The prospect of actually finding the funds to get to MD Anderson was a bit daunting. Aware of our finances, my uncle made the most gracious offer of sacrifice that anyone has ever made for me. With tears in his eyes, he admitted that he didn't have a lot of money, but he did have land, and he would willingly sell it to help me get the care that I needed for me and the baby. Stunned, I didn't know what to say. Here he sat ready to give up all he had for me and my family. It was the most touching gesture that I have ever experienced and one that I will never forget.

Finally, the day came that my children were coming to the hospital to see me. I was so excited! I thought they would never arrive. Upon entering my room, they seemed a bit frightened, not sure of what to expect. With Bobby's help, I pulled myself out of the bed, brushed my hair, straightened my gown, and forced a smile in an attempt to ease their fears. The nurse granted me permission to accompany them to the cafeteria for lunch. Although I was still not able to eat anything other than graham crackers and peanut butter, it filled me with joy just to be with them. The children quietly picked at their food. They were clinging to Dad, searching for the assurance that Mom was going to be all right.

We went back up to my floor, and finding a table in a nearby waiting room, we played a card game, Uno. I was so exhausted, I could hardly think straight. The pain was hammering me with full blows. I fought hard to hide it. I did not want them to leave, not without me. The time passed too quickly. It was getting late, and I was so weak, I could hardly stand. The time had come for them to go home—without me. I walked to the end of the hall to say good-bye. Emma grabbed onto my gown, crying and holding tight. Bobby had to pry her away from me. She was holding her arms out to me, begging me with her eyes to let her stay as Bobby continued walking down the hall carrying her away. Luke was crying also, and Jonathan, too old to cry in public, looked uneasy. They wanted me, and I wanted to be with them just as badly. With tears flowing freely down my cheeks, I watched through the window in the door until they were out of sight. I collapsed on the floor of the hall in a heap of sobs, feeling that my heart would burst from the pain as my grief and fatigue overcame me. I wanted to go home! They needed me, and I needed to be with them. The nurse helped me back to my room where I wept until I finally fell asleep. Upon awakening, I had a new determination to get home. I determined to get up and walk. Many times a day, during the next few days, I got up and walked the halls of the hospital, trying to gain strength enough to get home. Home was the prize on which I was keeping my focus.

No Place Like Home

After ten days in the hospital, it was my Luke's birthday. It was February 19, 2010, and my little boy was turning six years old. It was time for me to go home. Afraid that Bobby would object, I got a nurse to help me shower while he had gone to eat breakfast. I slowly and carefully put my things in my bag, put my tennis shoes on, and waited for the doctor. I was sitting on the bed with my feet propped up on my suitcase waiting when my surgeon, Dr. Calvin, came to my room finding me dressed, packed, and ready to leave. He walked in, looked at me, and asked, "Going somewhere?" To which I replied that I was going home. I was determined to get home for my baby's birthday, even though he was not a baby anymore. Seeing the determination behind my intention, Dr. Calvin consented and allowed me to be discharged. I was finally going home!

May 11, 1998, I was in a car accident that left it difficult for me to ride with others. It may be, perhaps, even more difficult for those who choose to drive with me in the car. I was hit head-on by a teenage boy who was passing a truck illegally in a dangerous curve. This accident wrecked more than just my car, it wrecked me psychologically. I travel much better behind the wheel, feeling that I am in control of the car. My very loving and understanding husband patiently allows me to do most of the driving.

As we were leaving the hospital, it became clear to me that there was absolutely no possible way that I would be allowed to drive. To argue would be pointless. So with Bobby's help, I climbed into the passenger's seat of the truck. The drive home took about fifty minutes. During this time, I never screamed, gasped, or told my husband how to drive. Amazing! I wasn't even scared. As I contemplated this change in me, the first thing to come to mind was the drugs. Guessing that I might be a bit sedated yet, I chalked it up to an unclear mind. However, as I contemplated further, I realized that I was no longer afraid of dying in an automobile accident. I had discovered that God didn't need an automobile accident to take me. He had cancer! The truth of it though is that God doesn't need cancer to take me either. God has a plan. It does not matter whether it is a car wreck, cancer, a heart attack, or any other means. God will call when he calls. He will come get me in his perfect time, not one second too soon nor one second too late. God used my cancer to give me freedom from fear and to remind me of what Jesus said in Matthew 6:27, "Who of you by worrying can add a single hour to his life?" I can live my life, without fear, knowing that God is in control.

Immediately after my diagnosis, but before surgery, my church family had lifted me up in prayer. It was the Sunday morning following my diagnosis. As soon as the pastor had given the invitation, I hurried to the front, where, lying on the altar, I pleaded with God to heal me. Seeing me kneeling up front, Pastor Todd took a moment to let our church family know that I was pregnant and had been diagnosed with cancer. I heard gasps echoing throughout the church. Members of the congregation began to move to the front joining me there for a time of prayer. Our pastor laid his hand upon my head as others gathered around to lay hands on me. He began to pray for God's healing on me. He concluded this prayer by praying that God's will be done. In that very moment, I glanced up at him as he stood over me and thought, *Buddy, you had better be sure it* is *God's will to heal me if you are going to pray like that.* I was not, quite frankly, interested in God's will at that time unless it was God's will to heal me. I quickly dismissed my concerns because I had already had a word from God and expected him to heal me. However, upon arriving home from the hospital that prayer began to haunt me. In light of what the doctors were now telling me, I was no longer sure that it was God's will to heal me.

Sick! I was sick! Physically, emotionally, I was barely surviving. Day after day, I lay on the couch. The emotional pain of listening to my life carry on without me as I continued to lay there, not being able to get up was almost unbearable! With every ounce of strength that I had, I made it to the shower. There, sitting on a stool as the water washed over me, I wept. It was the only place that I had where I could cry unhindered. I sobbed. My children couldn't hear. It was very difficult to try to hide my fears from my children. They asked me if I was going to die. I didn't know. Not wanting to lie to them, but not wanting to be honest either, I really didn't know what to say. They seemed distant from me as if they were afraid of me. I tried to reach out to them with the little strength I could muster to offer them a nugget of normalcy. Yet they carried on without me.

Bobby and I now found ourselves facing the biggest problem we had ever faced. I had cancer. I wanted to talk about it. I wanted to go over and over everything that had happened. I had a lot of questions. Having little memory of my time in the hospital, I wanted Bobby to give me play-by-play blows to fill in the gaps in my mind. Maybe I had hoped that if we kept at it long enough, we would come up with a way to make it not real. Bobby knew just how real it was, and he could not talk about it. This was one problem that he could not fix, and he saw no point in talking. Talking did not help him, it hurt him. I realized that I needed a friend, someone who would just listen to me talk, while feeling no obligation to me. I felt so isolated and alone. There was no one.

There was no one to take me by the hand and tell me that things would be all right. No one to reassure me by saying that they had been there and survived it. I had no one with whom I could relate. My situation was so rare! I often felt frustrated when well-meaning people proposed to think that they knew how I felt. Until you have been there, you cannot possible know what it feels like to be pregnant, have cancer, and have the responsibility of a family. I got so weary from hearing things like "you need your rest," "you need to take care of yourself," "don't try to do too much." I was the only one who could decide what I could and could not do. I often felt oppressed by the insistence of some that I needed to lay down or that I was trying to do too much. Only I could find the balance for me. Determined and seeking purpose, I needed to do as much as I was able.

My mother had been spending her days at my house, helping to care for household chores and to see after the children when I could not. My determination was never far from me. Desperate to get my life back, I claimed a strength that I did not really feel. I sent Bobby to work and told my mom that I was ready to try to make it a day on my own. Knowing me as well as she does, she surely felt that there was no point to argue. She probably also knew that I would never make it. Not yet. Still I told her to enjoy her day doing something for herself. I was going to take care of things on this day. Knowing what likely would be coming, she went home to wait.

The day started rather slowly. I was still struggling with morning sickness on top of everything else, but I managed to make it through breakfast. That was easy. The dishes in the dishwasher were clean, so the children could get clean bowls out of the dish washer. Jonathan was tall enough to reach the cereal and set it on the table. Luke got the milk out of the refrigerator. Emma got out spoons. Working together, they fixed their own cereal for breakfast. I happily sat on the couch, listening. By 10:30 a.m., things had taken a definite turn for the worse. Jonathan was sick. Luke had decided to make himself chocolate milk. I was napping on the couch, so he didn't want to disturb me. His adventure ended with an entire container of Nesquick being knocked over and off the table. I awoke to find my kitchen floor covered in chocolate milk mix. Luke and Emma were playing in it. Then there was the issue of the golf ball that had somehow found its way into the commode. Surveying the situation, I requested that someone please bring me the phone. Too sick to get up, I lay waiting. Phone in hand, I quickly dialed Mom's number. My explanation was simple. I had been wrong. No matter how badly I wanted to, I still was not strong enough to handle things on my own. "Come quickly!" I cried. My mother, living next door, arrived within minutes. She came in, looked around briefly before asking where I wanted her to start. I really did not care. I suggested perhaps the golf ball would be a good starting place being that I was nauseated and was uncertain how long it would be before I needed that commode. I lay quietly on the couch, listening as my mom went into the bathroom to fish out the golf ball as only a grandmother would do. As she was washing the ball, I heard her ask Emma, "Honey, when did you put the golf ball in the commode?" Emma cheerfully answered, "Right after I tee-teed." I lost the battle I was fighting and laughed out loud. With only one dirty look from my mom, mission number 1 was accomplished. Bless my mother's heart! My mom paused only for a moment. Then it was on to the kitchen to solve the next crisis. Through only the love of a grandmother did she find strength to endure.

One bright and sunny Sunday morning, I felt the strongest need to get to God's house. My family church is across the road from my house. It is a small country church where people come as they are and are received and loved. My husband helped me get dressed. With no makeup, make-shift maternity clothes, and tangled hair, I made it to the car, across the road, and into the church. When I walked through the door, the preacher stopped the service to welcome us. I was greeted with hugs and a genuine gladness to see me. As I sat in the pew feeling the love of family and friends, I fought back tears. How very grateful I was for the prayers of these people. It was humbling to me that they gave of their time to pray for me.

I never heard a word the pastor said that day. My thoughts were far from that place. I sat in the pew with my heart singing, "When we all get to heaven what a day of rejoicing that will be. When we all see Jesus, we'll sing and shout the victory." I felt God's presence. His assurance of heaven surrounded me. I gazed out of the church window across the cemetery and began to decide in which spot I might like to be buried. I was never afraid of dying; the thought of being with Jesus is exciting! Yet I was terrified of not being there for my children when they needed me. My tears were for my children. It was for them that I sat in church that Sunday morning pleading with God to let me live.

The community continued to reach out to our family with love and support. We were covered in prayers and love. Family members, church members, and friends were used by God to provide for our physical and spiritual needs. We had every meal prepared for us with love for about two months. We had financial gifts given to us out of love that covered the loss in my husband's pay checks almost to the penny. Prayer—it was the most coveted of gifts.

One afternoon as I lay on the couch, a knock sounded at the door. Doing a quick survey of the living room to determine my level of embarrassment at the clutter, I hesitantly asked my mom to answer the door. It was a beautiful angel of a lady who had heard about my situation and had come to offer prayer with us. After she prayed, she looked me in the eye and told me how she truly believed that I was going to be all right. She will never know the level of encouragement and comfort she brought to me. She also assured me that there were people all over the world that she had contacted, praying for me.

When my husband returned to work, he too was encouraged by strangers. A man at the gas pump stopped him to ask if he was the guy whose wife was sick. He wanted to pray with Bobby. Such was the scenario at restaurants, job sites, and throughout the county. We have never so been touch by the love of strangers, God's people, in our lives.

The Children

My darling children began to manifest their anxieties surrounding us and our present situation. These children were accustomed to a mom who had always been very active and involved with them. I had been their mom, teacher, cook, nurse, laundry maid, playmate, and their number one fan. Mom, as they had always known her, had ceased to be.

Emma was the youngest. At four years old, she was least able to verbalize her feelings. She became very clingy. Anytime I had to leave her sight, she would cry, desperately afraid that I would not come back. The ten days that I had been away at the hospital recuperating had seemed like an eternity to such a young child.

Luke, who was just turning six, was big enough to be sure that he was no baby, yet young and tender and desperately needing the assurance of his mom. He began to cry in the evenings. He was never able to pinpoint exactly why he was crying. So young, he was unable to really put his fears into words.

Jonathan, the oldest, was ten years old. Jonathan has always been a very responsible and sensitive young man. He took on much of the responsibility of the other children, fighting to keep a sense of normalcy. Driven by a deep loyalty to me, he was determined that nothing changed and became angry when others tried to help if they didn't do things the same way Mom did them.

Evidence of the depths of the children's anxiety became apparent one evening as I lay again on the couch. My mom had made a sandwich for Jonathan. Displeased that he was being asked to eat yet another sandwich and longing for Mom and the meals he was accustomed to, his attitude took a turn for the worse. Luke, seeing the disgruntled attitude leaking out of his brother, commented to Jonathan that he must be nice to grandmother. If he didn't keep on Grandmother's good side, Luke—ever the logical child—concluded, there would be no one to make their sandwiches when Mama died. Hearing this conversation was like being sucker punched in the gut! The pain in my heart was searing. I wanted so desperately to cook supper for my family! I wanted to do my job! I love washing their clothes and dishes. I love taking care of them. I find being a keeper of my home to be the most rewarding job in the world. It was killing me inside to have to let others do my job.

I had not realized how much my children had internalized. By not being more frank with them, I had allowed them to make their own assumptions as to what was happening. That was wrong of me. It really did more harm than good and did not protect them from anything. It was time to have an honest conversation with my children. Although I still did not have the answers that they sought, I understood that they needed to be a part of the process. Cancer is a family sickness, not an individual sickness. My entire family was a victim of this illness, and we needed to work through things as a family.

The conversation that I had overheard between Jonathan and Luke was truly a game changer for me. I realized that for weeks I had been laying on the couch, waiting to see how soon I would die. It came to my conscious attention that I wasn't dead yet, and it was time to get up! Realizing that I had been waiting to die motivated me to get up and fight to live. I went outside to sit in the sunshine, soaking up its rays. It felt so good, warming me to the bone. It seemed to be recharging me as a battery needs to be recharged. I began to feel alive. I started to walk. Although I didn't make it far that first day, it was a start. The next day, I walked a little farther, each day gaining more strength.

I made two doctor's appointments that day. The first was to see the ob-gyn. It occurred to me that I really did not know what condition the baby was in, if he was even still alive. After discovering that I had been given numerous drugs during and after my surgery that were incompatible with pregnancy, I needed to know if the baby had survived. The second appointment that I made that day was to see the oncologist. I had been left with many questions and few answers. I needed answers. I had to know what options might be available to me, but more importantly, I needed to know how long I had left to live.

The day came to visit Dr. Wolf. I had not seen him or spoken with him since being released from the hospital. As I waited in the exam room for him to come in, I prayed, begging God to let this baby be alive. Dr. Wolf entered the room and came directly to me to embrace me in a sympathetic hug. His words were few. Immediately, turning the monitor away from my view so as to spare me the distress of what he expected to find, he began the ultrasound that would reveal the condition of my baby.

Upon beginning the ultrasound, he commented that what he was seeing was the one thing that he had feared. I felt sick, so sure that my baby was dead. Dr. Wolf then continued by saying that my baby was perfectly healthy. I was confused. What had he feared? How did fear compute with my baby being perfectly healthy? My question was answered as he followed up by saying to me, "I had prayed that your baby would be dead when you got here today." I looked at him with astonishment and utter disbelief as he continued to tell me that he was as pro-life as anyone but that God had given medical doctors the knowledge for dealing with these types of situations. It was my duty and responsibility as a mother to abort and live.

Nausea began to creep up as I bit back the urge to vomit. He continued to reiterate what I had been told at the hospital, guaranteeing me that I would be dead within months if I tried to continue this pregnancy. Motioning toward Emma, who had accompanied me to the appointment, he asked me if I really wanted that little girl to grow up without her mama. Did I really want to leave my children as orphans, because if I tried to continue this pregnancy, that would be exactly what I was doing. He explained to me just how selfish it was of me to leave three children without a mother just to deliver a baby that would never even know me. And what about my husband? How unfair it was of me to leave my husband to raise four children alone. As I began to sob, he placed his arm around me and continued to explain that I had a week to have the "termination." If I did not do this right away, the procedure would be bloody, dangerous, and possibly fatal. Having grown weary from his hounding, I got up to leave. Leaving behind only the mascara stains on his shirt, I left his office never intending to return.

As I drove home from this appointment, I was distraught beyond anything I have ever experienced. Jonathan was riding in the seat behind me. Seeing my distress, he kept asking me if the baby was okay. It was the same question but phrased differently over and over. Jonathan is tenderhearted. He loves children and had been heartbroken over the loss of my previous pregnancies. As he continued to talk, I felt as if I would explode. I wanted to yell at him that it was not the baby that going to die, it was me. I couldn't, of course, say that to him. I needed to pull over. I needed to get out of the car and run, run away from this pain. I could hardly breathe, my chest hurt. *God*, I prayed, *please just help me get home.*

My mind continued to swirl. Why was God letting this happen to me? To my children? Was it something that I had done, or not done, that God was punishing me for? What in the world would become of them? I knew that my husband would always be a good dad, but to be perfectly honest, he is no Mr. Mom! As I continued to drive, I realized something that I am most ashamed to even admit. I realized that I had been expecting that the baby would be dead, that God would take this burden from me by his own hands and allow me the opportunity to fight for my life. God had already taken two of my babies. Why didn't he take this one so that I could live? Oh! The many times that I have asked God to forgive me for my lack of faith.

This was the beginning of the worst night of my life. When I got home, I went straight to the bathtub. Filling the tub with the hottest water I could stand, I laid back against the tub, closed my eyes, and placed a bath cloth over my face. This was the only place that I could go to grieve. The children were always watching me, and I needed to be strong for them. I had to hide or wait for them to go to sleep before I could release my real feelings and fears. As I lay in the bathtub with the bathroom door locked, I sobbed. I cried as my heart sang a song that I remembered from my childhood. It was a song that I recall having always comforted me in times of trouble. The words were "When I think I'm going under, part the waters, Lord. When I feel the waves around me, calm the sea. When I cry for help, oh hear me, Lord, and hold out your hand. Touch my life, still the raging storm in me." This song, I recalled hearing sang by Evie, brought me comfort. I sang it over and over in my heart, lying in the tub until the water had turned cold. I got out of the tub, wrapped up in whatever I could find, and called my aunt.

My aunt is an administrator at a hospital in a fairly large city. She had taken a faxed copy of my pathology report to some of the doctors that work at her hospital. The idea was to get a second opinion without my having to travel. I called her with the expressed purpose of tattling on Dr. Wolf for having been so cruel to me. She listened without a word. As I finished pouring out my distress, she calmly and softly answered, "Honey, Dr. Wolf is right." The doctors that she had conferred with were in agreement. They too believed abortion was my only option. My aunt promised to support whatever decision that I made, but it was clear to me that she was scared for me. The choice was mine to make, but I had to understand the consequences that I was leaving my family to face.

Being a Christian and having surrounded myself with Christian friends, I would have expected to be judged had I chosen to have an abortion. I was not prepared for being judged for choosing to have my baby. To be sure, it is hard to know what one might do in a situation without having been in that situation. Had I been on the outside looking into someone else's life, I too may have judged. Who knows? It was extremely painful, however, when our Christian friends, the ones we respect as people who love God, encouraged us to abort. There was very little support for us. Many came against me believing that the sacrifice of one baby outweighed the leaving behind of three. There was much fear for a husband who was burdened beyond what many believed he could bear. Others shared no opinion but came offering prayers and assistance. There were few who encouraged us by supporting our decision. I can count on one hand—make that a couple of fingers—the number of people that told us we were doing the right thing. Most promised prayer, but few took a stand.

The Valley of the Shadow

This evening, supper had been provided by friends. It was still warm, sitting on the stove. Bobby had only to put food on the plates, the plates on the table, and call the children in to eat. Being the mom, I never had to ask my children what they would like to eat. I know that Luke and Emma want the chicken leg. Jonathan likes the breast and wants mashed potatoes. Luke prefers macaroni. Emma drinks apple juice, milk for Luke, and tea for Jonathan. This is all just part of being mom. Bobby called the children to the kitchen where he made a royal error in judgment. He asked one collective question, "What do y'all want to eat?" I held my breath as "y'all" began answering all at once. During the erupting chaos of three children talking at one time, I took the opportunity to point out to God just how badly my family needed me.

With supper finished and the children dressed for bed, I lay on the bed listening as my husband began putting the children to bed. Quietly, I waited for everyone to fall asleep so that I could cry—alone. I didn't want to upset the children, and I didn't want to upset Bobby. This night was different than the rest. In Genesis, the Bible tells of God wrestling with Jacob.

Well, call me Jacob because God got with me this night. God began to call me in an almost audible voice. He called me to surrender. I agreed under the condition that God let me have my way—to heal me. I spent hours explaining to God that he must let me live. God told me to trust him. I cried. I prayed. I planned my funeral. I cried, I prayed, I began to plan what I would say to my children on my deathbed. I was most afraid that they would become angry with God for taking their mom. I needed to find the right words to say to them so that I could be sure that each one of them would choose to accept Jesus as Lord and Savior. Still, God was calling me to a place of surrender. Still, I refused. I continued to plan what nugget of truth and wisdom I could leave with each child. My prayer and hope was only that this child of mine would grow into the young adult of whom I had dreamed. Yet God was calling.

Weary and utterly exhausted, I lay across the bed, barely able to breathe. God spoke. God grabbed me by the heart and squeezed.

I heard him say, "You can trust me."

"But my children need me," I began to argue.

God answered, "No, they don't need you. They have me. Don't you understand that I created these children? I love them even more than you can fathom. I have a plan for them, a purpose for them, and I am all they need." God reminded me of his promise in Jeremiah 29:11 (NIV) for my children. "For I know the plans that I have for you declares the Lord, plans to prosper you and not to harm you, plans to give you hope and a future."

God was showing me that these are his children. I am just the childcare provider to whom he has entrusted them. The issue was not whether I lived or died, but rather did I trust God for my children. Would I surrender my will? Would I surrender my right to be their mom? Did I trust that if God took me from here he had something even better than me for them? Yes. I did. I finally understood that God was going to take care of my babies with or without me. In the early hours of the morning, as day was beginning to break, I raised my eyes toward heaven and gave up my life. I surrendered to God. For the first time, I had a peace that began to relieve me. In trusting God, my struggle was gone.

The Bible tells us in Psalms 30:5 (NIV), "Weeping may remain for a night, but rejoicing comes in the morning." The next morning was my first appointment with my oncologist, Dr. Stone. On the way to the appointment, all I could do was pray for peace. I expected the worst. Bobby and I sat outside the office before my appointment and prayed. We asked only for hope. I had become obedient to God's call to surrender, and he was about to birth that new hope in me.

As we sat in the waiting room filling out the new patient information sheets, I looked around. I didn't belong here. I was a young mother, not to mention with child. Everything seemed surreal. As I continued to sit on the couch in that waiting room, feeling very out of place, a tall fellow wearing a cowboy hat had noticed the blue new patient forms on which I was working. He approached me to inquire about my circumstances. I quickly learned that cancer patients have a community of their own. They love and support one another with an understanding that only they share. It is an exclusive club that one can only become a member of when he or she too becomes a victim. So this club member approached me asking about the type of cancer that I had. He shared about his own battle with cancer. He then instructed my husband to buy me a nice hat, preferable a cowboy hat. He leaned closer, looked Bobby in the eye, and declared in a raspy voice, "When it gets so bad that she can't stand it, get her some marijuana. If she is too sick to smoke it, brew it and let her drink it." Only one thing was going through my mind at that point. I was terrified at the suffering that this man believed I was facing. The nurse called my name, and as I gathered my things to go meet with the doctor, this same man in the cowboy hat stopped me. He quickly asked if I knew God and would I pray for him. I agreed. Many nights I have prayed for that man. I have not seen him since that day.

Ray of Hope

Once in the patient room, we waited. My body and mind were numb as I waited. *God*, I whispered in my heart, *I can't bear any more.* I remembered that God had promised in his word not to allow more on me than I could bear. I was reminding God of that promise when in walked Dr. Stone. Getting straight to the point, he faced me as he inquired as to my decision concerning the baby. I explained to him that I was having this baby. I would like very much to live, but I was definitely having this baby. You could have heard a pin drop as we waited for his reply. He quickly and simply said, "Okay." *"Okay" to which part?* I wondered. Then as he began to explain that he thought it was possible to save both me and the baby, my husband and I looked at each other with total disbelief.

Dr. Stone went on to explain that he had seen a pregnant woman with breast cancer receive chemotherapy. The mother and baby had done fine. This, of course, was not breast cancer, but he felt the same chemotherapy drugs would be appropriate. He did not make me any promises, but he was willing to treat me. He was willing to take a chance on me when other doctors pressured him not to treat me. I would soon learn the extent of the prophetic provision that God had made for me concerning this particular doctor.

When my diagnosis was made, the hospital issued a routine call to the cancer center to request a consultation with an oncologist on my behalf. Dr. Stone was on call this particular day. Having only been practicing in our area for a short time, he had spent the past several years working at one of the world's leading cancer institutions, MD Anderson, in Houston. My plans had been to go to MD Anderson to research possible treatment options, but God brought MD Anderson to me. While Dr. Stone was still in Houston, MD Anderson was conducting a study on pregnant women with breast cancer, and the results had been positive. Having been a witness to this research, Dr. Stone was the perfect match for me. God put the perfect doctor in our path, giving us our first ray of hope.

I stepped out of Dr. Stone's office into the warmest, brightest sunlight that I have ever felt. The air smelled so fresh. The grass and trees were so green. I felt God's presence surrounding me. I knew in that moment that I was going to live.

> You turned my wailing into dancing;
> You removed my sackcloth and clothed me with joy,
> that my heart may sing to you and not be silent.
> O, Lord my God, I will give you thanks forever.
>
> Psalms 30: 11-12 NIV

Upon arriving home that afternoon, a dear friend called to tell me that she felt God leading her to give me a new verse. She challenged me to get my Bible and read John 11:4 (NIV). John 11:4 states, "This sickness will not end in death. No, it is for God's glory so that God's son may be glorified through it." As I began to read through John chapter 11, God began to reveal his purpose to me.

In chapter 11 of the book of John, a man named Lazarus dies. This is a man that Jesus loved. Jesus received word that Lazarus was sick, yet he remained where he was for two more days. How hard it must have been for Martha and Mary to understand why Jesus did not come immediately. Lazarus had died by the time Jesus arrived. Why had Jesus allowed this to happen? The answer is simple. This was the way that God got the most glory. By allowing Lazarus to die, Jesus' power was revealed as he raised Lazarus from the dead.

My vision became clear as I could see that God was purposing his will for my life that he might be glorified. God had promised to heal me from the very beginning, but not understanding his plan, I had given to doubt. I began to recognize that yes, God certainly could have healed me on the operating table just as he could have healed Lazarus when he was sick. But that wasn't the way that God could get the most glory. How easy it would have been to recognize what a wonderful surgeon that I'd had, who had gotten out all my cancer. My story would have ended, and I would have had a much less effective testimony. God chose this path for me so that others could see his power. And yes, he loves me. He chose me because he loves me.

It was decided by my oncologist that I was to start chemotherapy at fourteen weeks' gestation. I was extremely nervous at the prospect, but I knew that I really didn't have a choice. My surgeon scheduled an appointment for me to receive the dreaded port. I was terrified, for some unexplainable reason, to have my port placed. Other survivors reassured me that it was a simple procedure, not to be feared. One very special friend, Chandler, became my most solid supporter. As a survivor himself, he was able to walk me through the unknown and comfort me in a way that others could not. He assured me that the port would be my friend. Seeing no alternative, I showed up for my appointment to have the procedure that would place a port-a-catheter into my chest. This would provide an easy access point for the chemo that I was to receive and protect my veins from the harsh drugs that were to be administered.

The procedure went well, just as Chandler had assured me it would—simple, quick, and painless. Immediately following the insertion of the port, I was taken to recovery where I would remain until the anesthesia began to wear off. This became my favorite part of all the procedures that I was to endure. That blessed relaxed state of existing where reality is hours away from crashing back down around me—just for a few moments, to forget the truth of my circumstances.

As I was coming out of numb oblivion, I looked up and quite by accident made eye contact with Dr. Wolf. What in the world was he doing here? This was the recovery room at the hospital. It was one of those moments where he saw me at the same time that I saw him. It wasn't as if we could pretend that we hadn't seen each other. He stepped closer to ask me what I was doing here. I, in somewhat slurred speech, informed him that I had just had my port placed. He stood looking at my belly with the obvious question. He never asked, he didn't have to, I volunteered that yes, I was indeed still pregnant. A little better than three months to be exact, and I was to start chemotherapy the next day. He looked at me hard as he inquired as to whom had told me that this was safe. I assured him that I had every confidence in Dr. Stone. Dr. Wolf then logically pointed out to me that either he was right in telling me that what I was about to do would kill me and the baby, or Dr. Stone was right in his opinion that I could have chemo while pregnant, live, and have a healthy baby, but one of them had to be wrong. I had better be sure that I made the right choice about who to believe—my life depended on it. Speech still slurring, I assured him that God was taking care of me. Without another word, he gave me the thumbs up sign as if to say I have tried to warn you; then he turned and slowly walked away.

The following morning came too quickly. This was the big day, the day that I was to begin taking chemotherapy. As

I prepared to leave for this appointment, I packed a bag that had been lovingly given to me by a lady from our church. It was to be my "chemo bag" and later became Joshua's diaper bag. It had been packed for me with a blanket, pack of tissues, lotion, hand sanitizer, and Chap Stick. I added a few snacks and some reading material. With that, we were out of the door.

The drive to the doctor's office was filled with trepidation. I tried not to think of all that could go wrong. I was concerned, first, about the baby. I was also very concerned about how sick this poison was going to make me. I was terrified of becoming bedridden, missing an entire year of my children's lives. That may seem ridiculous, considering that I had been facing the likelihood of missing the rest of my children's lives. Still, a year is a long time, and I was scared of how badly I might suffer from the effects of the chemotherapy. The very idea of chemotherapy went against me. The whole concept of pouring poison into my veins was difficult to swallow. I am a fairly health-conscious person. We grow a good bit of our own food, organically, and I buy organic whenever available. We can and preserve as much of our homegrown vegetables and herbs as possible. What I was about to do felt contrary to healthiness, yet this seemed to be the best, if not the only, option for me.

Upon arriving at the doctor's office, I had a quick weigh in followed by a blood draw. Now it was time to get started. The nurse quickly accessed my port. Ouch! At least it was quick. I began this treatment as well as every subsequent treatment with prayer, first, for my baby's safety, and then for the chemotherapy to kill the cancer in my body. It was now time to get started. The nurse first hooked me up to a bag of Zofran to lessen, if not eliminate the nausea that was to follow. It didn't work! As the Zofran poured into my body, I sat very still, afraid to move. Just lifting my head to look up made me dizzy. I hoped this feeling would pass quickly. It was unnerving, yet I told no one. I didn't want to do anything that might slow my treatment down; it was already going to be a long day, and I was anxious to return home to my children. Next up was a bag of steroids, followed by Leucovorin. The Leucovorin was given to help the 5-FU to work more effectively. I was then given a pump to disperse the chemotherapy drug 5-FU through my body. This pump would infuse the drug into my body for twenty-two hours, at which time the pump would be removed. Four hours after beginning, I was finished with treatment number one. It would be two weeks before the process would be repeated.

The cancer support center in our area was a place of refuge. I turned to them for information on research, reading materials including children's books about having a parent with cancer, and many other forms of support. One measure of support that they offer is wigs and turbines for those beginning chemotherapy. After looking up the specific chemo drugs that

I would be receiving, the nurse explained that my hair would likely fall out by about the third treatment. I could expect a tingling feeling on my scalp, and then one day the hair would begin to come out by the clumps. The cancer center gave me a wig to keep with me at home in preparation for losing my hair. Not a natural blond, I laughed when I was given a long blonde wig. Maybe blondes do have more fun.

Following the advice of other survivors who had already been through treatments, I had my hair cut short. The idea was that losing my hair would not be such a shock if it was already short. Remaining positive, I amused myself by considering how quickly I could get ready for church when all that I had to do was to wash my head and put my hair on with my clothes. Trying to keep things light for the children, I modeled the wig for them, pretending that I thought it was really cool. Emma wanted a turn. Putting the wig on, she ran to the mirror to check out her appearance. Continuing to keep the tone light, we suggested the boys take a turn. Laughter filled the room as Jonathan and then Luke tried on the wig. Nothing was more hilarious however, than when it was their dad's turn. Now, to be sure, I find my husband to be an attractive fellow, but seeing him in that blond wig was frightening. I had a flashback to the long-haired rockers of the eighties. Yikes!

Lucky for me, Emma had prayed every night during my treatments that God would not let mommy's hair fall out.

How grateful I am that God used that opportunity to show this little child his willingness to affirm her prayer, and my hair never fell out.

With each treatment, I pleaded with God to keep my baby safe. I would pray for him to show me his hand in this, to confirm that he was taking care of Joshua. After Emma was born, Bobby and I were certain that there would be no more children for us. I had gotten rid of all baby items. We didn't have as much as a sippy cup left in our house. As I continued to pray for God's assurance concerning the baby, he began to move. After each treatment, as I prayed, my phone would ring. Each time, it would be someone offering baby items. Over the course of my treatments, every single item that we needed for the baby was offered to us on loan or as a gift. Finally, after several months, I began to get what God was telling me. He was in control and was taking care of Joshua. I had absolutely nothing to worry about. God wasn't going to provide everything we needed to take care of a baby if he was just going to snatch him away. God has provided everything that Joshua has needed as he has needed it. At eight months old, I still have not had to buy as much as a diaper.

Along with beginning chemotherapy, it was time to find an ob-gyn. Dr. Wolf had asked that I at least talk to a specialist. His office secured for me an appointment with Dr. Rose.

Many times I nearly backed out of keeping this appointment. I was not prepared to have yet another doctor promising me certain death if I continued my pregnancy. I was alone when I met with Dr. Rose. When his nurse called my name, I arose, following her down the hall and into his office where I was seated across from him. He was on the phone. I nervously wrung my hands as I waited. When he finally completed his telephone conversation, he introduced himself as he shook my hand. I wasted no time and made no bones. I simply informed him that if it was his intention to urge me to abort, then we were wasting his time and mine.

Surprise and relief washed over me as he explained that he was quite frankly puzzled at the urgency with which Dr. Wolf had felt it was necessary for me to abort. Dr. Rose had done some research, and he, like Dr. Stone, believed that my case was not hopeless. Dr. Rose was a specialist and would not be delivering my baby, but he promised to put me in touch with a real pro-life doctor. Yet again, God gave me new hope.

A few days later, Dr. Young called me to explain that Dr. Rose had contacted him about my case. He was honored and excited about the opportunity to support me in this pregnancy. He applauded my decision to choose life for my baby. Dr. Young arranged an appointment for me at his office. Upon meeting him for the first time, God confirmed for me that this was indeed the doctor that would help me get through this pregnancy. I sat in amazement as Dr. Young explained that he had done an internship at MD Anderson in Houston. Furthermore, his first name was Joshua. He prayed with me, encouraged me, and supported me in every possible way. I called him weekly seeking to come by the office and listen to the baby's heartbeat. He was glad to oblige. Anything that I needed to give me peace of mind, he graciously provided. That was all the confirmation that I needed from God to be sure that this was the right doctor.

From Denial to Acceptance

As I continued the chemotherapy, prayers were going up on my behalf from people I did not know and from places I have never been to. To be so completely covered in prayer is amazing and humbling. The chemotherapy wasn't as bad as I had feared. It was bad enough, but it wasn't completely debilitating, as I had feared.

As I progressed, still able to function, I went to this lovely place called denial. It occurred to me that if I didn't look sick and I didn't act sick, perhaps I wasn't really sick. Looking in the mirror I confirmed that I didn't look too bad, not as bad as I had seen others taking chemo look. In addition to looking halfway decent, I was still functioning, on some level at least. So I determined to not have cancer. I continued to home-school my children, manage our home, on some level anyway, and keep the children in their extracurricular activities. It was very important, I thought, to keep as much normalcy in our daily lives as possible. Although I still managed to stumble through daily life, there was nothing normal about it. I was doing everything that I could to keep things as they had been before my diagnosis, but nothing was the same. My efforts were a futile attempt in proving that I wasn't sick.

I realized the error of my thinking one day when, after my chemo treatment, I went home, picked up the children, and went to Wal-Mart to do some back-to-school shopping. Each of the three children had $30 to spend on the school supplies of his or her choice. As they made their choices, I struggled to keep up with who was getting what and how much each child's choices were adding up to. Finally, giving up in frustration, I announced that we had enough and it was time to go. If only there were words sufficient enough to describe my shock and confusion when the cashier announced that my total was in excess of $300! How in the world could that be right? I stood looking perplexed at the few bags of items that now lay in the buggy. What in the world could be in those bags? I could not remember! Not wanting my confusion to be obvious, I prayed that the check I was about to write would not bounce. I thought that I would get home and pick out the unneeded items to return for a refund.

My head was throbbing from the ensuing headache that I had developed during the drive home as I tried to remember what was in that buggy. When I came in, my husband was already home. Having found that sometimes it is easier to just come clean than to beat around the bush, I nervously announced that I had just blown $300 and had absolutely no idea what I had bought. Bobby stood looking stunned. I wasn't sure if it was the money or my irresponsibility that alarmed him the most. I began to cry, not to manipulate him into forgiving me, but because it sincerely scared me that my mind could be so blank. Anyone who has ever experienced chemo brain may be able to relate. It is frightening to be aware of what you should know but don't.

My independent streak can be a good thing, but it can also be not so good. On yet another occasion, I again determined to prove that I was not sick. Familiar with farm equipment, I find it to be relaxing and rewarding to work with the tractor. I had a brilliant idea. I would bushhog in the pasture and surprise Bobby when he got home from work. Surprised he was! With Jonathan reasonably suggesting that that was not a good idea, off I went. After only about fifteen minutes of driving the tractor, I hit something. This something did not sound good. Darn! I got off the tractor and raised the bushhog to find my husband's come-along tangled up in the blades. Double darn! As soon as he drove in, those big-mouthed kids of mine went running to tell Dad what mischief Mom had found. He quietly assessed the situation as I slunk back, waiting. Finally, he looked at me, and with the best Ricky Ricardo voice he could muster, he simply yelled "Lucy!" mimicking the 1960's hit show *I Love*

Lucy. He then suggested that in the future, when I wanted to help, the best help that I could be was to not help.

After that, I was banned from driving the tractor for the time being. All I had left to cause trouble with was the push mower. I actually enjoy doing yard work although you couldn't tell it by looking at my yard. I used mowing the grass as another attempt to prove that I was not sick, resenting anyone who dared to suggest that I shouldn't be cutting the grass. One night as I was mowing, I began to feel sick to my stomach. Unable to control the urge to vomit, I paused to take care of things and went right back to mowing. I was proud of myself thinking that I hadn't gotten caught until I looked up and saw Bobby running toward me from the field. Darn! I steeled myself for the coming explosion that insisted that I had no business mowing and I was to go inside at once.

Nevertheless, I was successfully, in my mind, proving that I was not sick. Things went from bad to worse when at my next appointment I had the audacity to suggest to Dr. Stone that I really did not have cancer after all. His response began with, "Lady, you have no idea how sick you are." He continued by suggesting that I quit whining about having treatments. He informed me that there were eighty-year-old women taking the same treatment that I was getting without complaint. Oh man, I was ticked! How dare he suggest that I did indeed have cancer. Besides, he did not understand that those eighty-year-old women didn't have a family for which they were responsible. They could have treatment and then go lie on the couch and watch TV for several days. I, on the other hand, had a life to lead. I left his office angry with a capital A.

Once we had gotten into the car to go home, my husband, knowing that I make jelly each year to give to family and friends for Christmas, queried, "So I guess he's off the jelly list?"

"Yep," I confirmed.

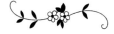

For weeks, friends and family had been encouraging me to register for the Relay for Life Survivor's Lap. Relay for Life is a fund-raising event to raise money for the research for a cure for cancer. It is also an organization that honors survivors. I had agreed that signing up for Relay for Life was something that I needed to do. Somehow, though, every time I drove toward the place to register, my car just kept going. I had told myself that I just wasn't as sick as all those other people with cancer. Therefore, it wouldn't be right for me to walk in the survivor's lap. However, after I had some time to consider what Dr. Stone had told me, I came to admit that I did indeed have cancer and that it would be a privilege for me to join together and walk with other cancer survivors in the Relay for Life. Finally, I mustered enough courage to sign up.

Our county chairperson works at the bank in town, so this was the location where I had to go to register. I slowly and hesitantly pulled into the bank parking lot. Sitting in the car for only a moment, I took a deep breath and mustered up enough courage to go inside. As I entered the bank, I felt nervous and awkward, unsure of what I was about to do. Ava, the county chairperson, spotted me. She knew who I was, though we had never met. Everyone in town seemed to know about the pregnant lady with cancer. She ushered me into her office. I sat down across from her at her desk, took a deep breath, and with a calmness that I did not feel, simply stated that I was here because I needed to register for the Relay for Life Survivor's Lap. After only a brief pause, I continued, "Because I have cancer." Hearing myself say that aloud took my breath away. I suddenly and uncontrollably began to sob. Ava quietly offered me a tissue. With tears pouring down my cheeks, I looked at her and said, "It's true, I really, really do have cancer." I continued to sit there in the quietness of the room contemplating that I really did have cancer. Although I had said it many times, I guess I never really had accepted it as truth. It was time for me to get real. My doctor had been right. I was a sick lady, and denying that truth was not healthy. I had to face my sickness and fight the illness, not the diagnosis.

A peace that doesn't even make sense came with the acceptance that I found that day, sitting in Ava's office at the bank. My coming experience with Relay for Life was touching. The support of my family was truly amazing. In preparation of the coming Relay for Life walk, my cousin Julie, along with Bobby, designed T-shirts unique to me and my circumstances. The shirts were cobalt blue, the color to represent colon cancer. They had a mother holding her baby on the front and the words "2 Survive." The back had the Bible verse John 11:4 printed on it. My entire family and extended family along with friends, bought these shirts to wear in support for me.

Because it is so difficult to find cancer ribbons in colors other than pink, my children and I bought cobalt-blue ribbon and made our own. We painted the word *survivor* on mine. As we were dressed and preparing to leave, my son Luke suggested that we pin a ribbon on my belly for Joshua. Joshua was, after all, already a big part of our family. At the relay event, I found a love among survivors that touched me in the depths of my soul. These were people who had walked where I was walking, with the exception of being pregnant, but they had made it. Nothing encouraged me more than to hear stories of survival of many years. Cancer did not always win! When the relay started, the survivors were assembled together to take the first lap. As we began to walk, supporters lined up around the track, clapping to show their support. It was an emotional moment in which I could not control the tears rolling down my face.

A Season for All Things under Heaven

As winter turned into spring, God gave me a new appreciation for the new life that springs forth each year. I had been through the winter in life and in season. Spring was bursting forth with new life just as I was bursting with new hope for life. I went outside daily to examine the progress of the trees and plants that were budding. I waited with excited expectation for the buds to open up into beautiful flowers. These buds represented my life. I was trusting God to let me bloom. For the first time in my life, I understood how my dear grandmother knew the names of every plant in her yard, and there were many. The connection between spring and the promise of new life no longer escaped me.

It was this same spring that my grandmother left this life to be with her Lord and Savior whom she dearly loved. She was excited to be with Jesus. There were times in sickness that she had gotten her hopes up that Jesus was on his way to get her. Those had not been her time, but she waited expectantly. Her time came on the same day that the doctor told us that

Joshua was indeed a boy, just as the Lord had told me he would be many months earlier.

The nurse who had been caring for my grandparents had called this particular morning with concern about my grandmother. She was confused and not responding as she normally would. Something was wrong. I had an appointment with Dr. Young that morning that I needed to keep. When he came into the exam room, I explained that I needed to get to my grandmother. Fearing the worst, I was in a rush. Dr. Young completed my exam in record time, revealing that the baby was a boy. Racing straight to my grandmother's house after my appointment, I was desperate to get to her before it was too late. Driving too fast, I prayed that God would grant that I might have the opportunity to spend just a few more moments with her. He did. God allowed me the privilege of spending the rest of the afternoon with my grandmother and gave me the opportunity to tell her that the doctor had confirmed that Joshua was a boy. I feel confident that she understood because she looked me in the eye, holding my gaze, as she nodded at me.

Spending that last afternoon with her was a priceless gift. I held her hand, looking at the fingers that had rubbed my feet to help me fall asleep when I was a child. These hands had taught me how to make biscuits and crab apple jelly. Most importantly, these hands had folded in prayer for me. Her greatest legacy was how she loved the Lord. That evening, she peacefully passed into her reward.

When I was a child, my great uncle passed away. Afraid of the body, I stayed far away from the casket at the funeral home. My grandmother, seeing my fear, came to sit with me. She explained to me that Uncle Carey was not here. This body that he had left behind was only a temporary house for his soul, a house that he no longer needed. God had given him a new one, a better one. Her explanation was comforting to me as we prepared to bury his old, empty house.

When my great-aunt Sarah passed away years later, I grieved so deeply. I felt sorry for myself and the loss that I was experiencing. Loneliness and sadness burdened me. But on this day, as I sat in the church at my grandmother's funeral, my perspective was different. After having stared death in the face myself, I had a new understanding and peace. I wasn't sad. I was celebrating, celebrating a life that had meant so very much to me and had touched me in so many ways. My grandmother was not dead; she was very much alive in her new house, a house that she could run and jump in without pain. She was with Jesus! I was so excited for her. The best part was the assurance that I would be with her again. The next time I got to be with her, which would be forever, we would never have to say good-bye again. She was alive in Christ. Her funeral was a time of excited praise. At her funeral, I wrote the following poem as if she were speaking to me.

Do Not Cry for Me

Do not cry for me
For I am not here, you see
I have gone ahead of you
To meet my Savior in eternity

Do not cry for me
For I am not here, you see
I have received my heavenly reward
Perfect healing, perfect love

So carry on in service
Until the Savior calls
Serving him with gladness
In love and with hope for all

Soon we'll meet again
On beautiful streets of gold
Our hope is in Christ Jesus
Our Savior to behold

So do not cry for me
I am already gone, you see
I wait for you with joy
To join me in eternity

Following the funeral service, family and friends came to the house to eat, reminisce, and share stories of a life well lived. I was sitting outside on the patio in the swing with my cousin Eric reminiscing about the summers we had spent at our grandmother's house when we were growing up, when we were approached by a lady who relayed to us that she had known of a woman, who like me, had been pregnant while having cancer. It was a woman who attended her church. This pregnant lady, we were told, also had several children and refused to abort the child that she was carrying. She and I apparently had much in common. Following the story closely, I then inquire of the child that this lady had been carrying. It had been two years, and the child was doing very well. I felt somewhat relieved until I followed up with the next logical question. I asked, "Well, how is the mom doing?" The answer shocked us all as this storyteller shared that the mother had passed away immediately following the birth of the baby. I sat in horror and shock. Eric looked as if he wanted to slug her for telling me such a story. I just wanted to throw up. Fear invaded my entire body. Satan took a front row seat in my mind, saying to me, "You see, you *are* going die." Silly me, I listened.

The story of this other mom plagued me. Satan told me that I was going to die, that my children were going to have horrible lives as orphans. I thought I had settled this, but Satan had gotten his foothold in my mind and was having a party. Several days of fretting past before I finally returned to the One in control. I got down on my knees one evening, having remembered that God had promised me healing, and I asked God to once again confirm for me that he had everything under control. In his loving-kindness, he spoke. As I was reading my evening devotional, the key verse for the night was Psalms 118:17. The Bible says in Psalms 118:17(NIV), "I will not die but live, and will proclaim what the Lord has done." Continuing to read, I found that this devotional passage had been written by a missionary who had been exposed to AIDS. She was awaiting test results to determine if she had in fact contracted the dreaded disease. God confirmed that he was definitely speaking to me when I got to the bottom of the passage to find that the missionary's name was Amy! I immediately woke my husband up as I was singing with relief, "I am *not* going to die." He sleepily replied, "I know, I thought we settled this a long time ago." Not to mention it was two o'clock in the morning.

I laid in bed still contemplating the verse that God had used to speak to me. I seemed to recall something about proclaiming. I got up, checked the verse again, and began to feel ill. What is this about proclaiming what the Lord had done? Not really caring that it was 2:00 a.m., I again woke my husband. "Honey, you don't think God would really make me stand up in front of people to tell what he has done for me, do you?" I asked timidly. My husband confirmed my worst fear with a simple word, "Yes."

Those who know me well know that this is not something that I would ever choose for myself. I am shy by nature. To illustrate just how uncomfortable I am in front of groups of people, allow me to share my Bible school experience. I love to teach Bible school. I love Jesus, I love children, and I love to teach. Bible school is the place to be for this perfect combination. I have always volunteered to teach, but it always came with one condition. On Friday night, when it was time to present the children with certificates for participation in VBS, someone else had to get up in front of the church to hand out the certificates for my class. Unless I had a volunteer lined up to hand out those certificates, I would not agree to teach. Yet here I was, being called by God to stand up in front of large groups of people to share what God had done for me. He had to be kidding. I patiently explained to God that Bobby was with me every step of this journey and that I would gladly support him as he stood up to tell our story. I call this my Moses moment. But God said no. It was my calling; no one else could do this for me. I knew that I was being called, but I also knew it wasn't time just yet.

Joshua's Tiny Cry

I was to have twelve chemotherapy treatments before giving birth. That was the goal. After eleven treatments, however, I began to have contractions that were strong enough to land me in the hospital. I hit my knees hard, praying once again for God's protection for Joshua. As excited as I was about meeting Joshua, I knew it was not time. At only thirty-two weeks, it was still too early. The nurses got the contractions to stop and sent me home with instructions to stay off my feet. Staying off my feet was easy. I was huge with pregnancy, and the August heat was hard for me to bear. Staying off my feet sounded like a good idea to me. Dr. Stone felt that it was time to stop chemotherapy until after the birth. The benefit of one last treatment did not outweigh the potential risk to the baby if he were to be born prematurely.

On August 28, 2010, I arrived at the hospital at 6:00 a.m. to have a scheduled C-section. This was the big day. The day we had been waiting for had finally arrived. I was surprised to find some of our friends already there awaiting Joshua's arrival. Unable to believe that they had beaten us to the hospital, I realized that they shared my excitement and anticipation about this special day. It was with great anticipation mixed with a bit of trepidation that I waited to be checked in.

Once we completed the check-in procedures, preparations began. Because I have rolling veins, starting the IV was usually the one of the hardest parts for me. Not this time. I had the port, one poke and I would be done. The maternity nurses didn't have any experience with a port-a-catheter, most never even having seen one. They called to the oncology floor to have a nurse sent up to access my port. Upon her arrival, the show began. Nurses, appearing to have come from everywhere, came by my room, requesting permission to watch. I was glad to grant that permission although I felt like an elephant in a circus with spectators coming from all around.

As the nurse finished preparing me for surgery, Dr. Young came into the room to speak to me. He asked that Bobby, and the others in the room, two of whom were pastors, gather around me to pray. It felt good to be surrounded by God's men. Dr. Young began praying as the prayer went from person to person around the circle. I felt God! He was with us in that room. Dr. Young then announced, "It's time." The wait was finally over. The time had arrived for us to meet this miracle growing inside of me. We said good-bye to friends as I was wheeled to the operating room.

Prior to surgery, Dr. Young had warned me of the possibility of my having to have a hysterectomy during surgery. This was my fourth C-section, raising the likelihood that I would have scarring that would make the surgery more difficult. Considering the fact that I had recently had colon surgery, he was concerned about what he would find when he cut me open. Therefore, it's understandable that he had scheduled extra time in the operating room in anticipation of possible complications. As he began the operation, he declared, "Well, this is another answer to prayer." Not sure what he was talking about, I inquired. He explained that there was little to no scarring from my previous C-sections nor my colon surgery. What a blessing! No complications or problems at all were encountered. The surgery continued. Within minutes, I heard the most beautiful sound that has ever filled my ears, my Joshua's tiny cry. He was here. He was alive. Everything looked normal. Everything was normal.

After having endured eleven chemotherapy treatments in utero, Joshua, which in Hebrew means "God saves" was born with no complications and no evidence of any exposure to chemotherapy. As soon as I was able to return to my hospital room, Joshua's siblings were brought in to meet their baby brother. They seemed surprised at how tiny our baby was. The arguing began immediately, with each one wanting a turn to hold the new baby. They didn't get much of a turn because visitors filled our room for most of the day. Some came to support us and share in our joy. Others came to see if this chemo baby would really be normal.

One week after Joshua was born, I returned to the cancer center for my final treatment of 5-FU, which had been postponed. For months, Joshua and I had fought this cancer battle together. His battle had been won, yet mine continued. Fear for Joshua's well-being during my previous treatments had been my primary concern, distracting me from any fear for myself. Concern for him gave me courage and strength to fight for us both. Now, separated from my son, I felt empty and alone. My courage wavered, yet I persevered. Once completed, I was then given four weeks to heal before I was to begin radiation.

I enjoyed the break from treatment, filling my days with time spent with my children and my new baby. During this time, my children got a glimpse of the mom they used to know. I was feeling better and becoming more active with them. Bobby was back at work full time, and things were beginning to have a more normal feel. I was cooking more, getting the house straightened out, and we were getting caught up on schoolwork. Structure returned to our home. The fog that I had been living in was lifting, and the children were thriving.

The day came too quickly for me to begin the next phase of treatment. I was to receive thirty-one treatments of radiation while taking the chemotherapy drug Xeloda. I was terrified. Covered in prayer, I began this new journey. It took almost an hour to drive to my daily radiation appointments, and then I had to make the trip home. I was to receive radiation daily, Monday through Friday, until I completed thirty-one treatments. The first week was uneventful. I went in, took my treatment, and left. I had some nausea from the Xeloda, and was tired from traveling, but overall, it was manageable.

As the treatments continued, I found them much more difficult to take. By the sixteenth treatment, I had already had all I could stand. Bowel movements were excruciating. The radiation had damaged my rectum, and the pain was searing. Bobby once told the doctor that he could measure my pain level by how loudly I screamed when I had to use the bathroom. Crying, I called the doctor to tell him that I could not stand any more. He asked me to come in to talk. I hesitated, fearing he might attempt to convince me to go ahead with my treatment that day; however, there was nothing he could have done to get me back in that machine at that time. I realized then, there were things that were worse than dying and this was one of them. Certainly, there must be radiation in hell.

Surprisingly, the doctor did not insist that I continue treatment. Rather, he suggested that I take a two-week break and then try to finish the rest of the treatments. I agreed in an attempt to stall an argument that I realized would be forthcoming with my husband because I had no real intention of ever returning. I kept asking God to let me stop. I knew without a doubt that he could cure me without the radiation. All I needed was affirmation from him that I didn't need to finish the treatments. I never got it. After much prayer and consideration, I did return to the radiologist to complete the last fifteen treatments. It was excruciating.

Many times, as I sat on the toilet screaming, my husband would get on his knees, lay his hands on me, and with tears running down his face, plead with God to help me. He begged God to let him take the pain for me. If I had ever doubted his love for me, I didn't now. It was obvious how it hurt him to see me in such agony. Eventually, thinking that if I didn't eat, I wouldn't need to use the bathroom, I quit eating. It didn't work. Surviving only on God's mercy and pain medications, I continued.

Having only one bathroom is tricky when a family member is as sick as I was. I was always in the bathroom. Playing charades once, I saw Emma ask the boys, "Who am I?" She then proceeded to run into the bathroom and start screaming.

The boys looked at me with deep concern. Emma was too young to understand, but Jonathan was deeply concerned that my feelings would be hurt. They were, but I would never let him know.

I looked at Emma, and with a counterfeit laugh to mask my true feeling, I exclaimed, "You sounded just like me!"

"Yep," she confirmed smiling.

Months later, while I was outside walking around with the children, Jonathan showed me a special place they had made. They thought that I might like to see the spot in the woods where they had built an outhouse while I was taking radiation. I was horrified and embarrassed. It saddened me to know that my sickness had forced them to go outside to use the bathroom.

Only by God's help did I finally finish the radiation. It was tough! I could only commit to one treatment at a time. As I left each day, sick as a dog, nauseated, and hurting, I told the nurse that I would probably be back tomorrow, but I was asking the question of myself, would I really come back? I never made it a promise. The possibility of ever going back was too painful and sickening to even contemplate that soon after a treatment. One day at a time, moment by moment was all I could face. Even as I walked down the hall to the treatment room, I was still unsure if I could make myself climb up on that table to be burned yet again. Dr. Stone had promised me that if I completed all thirty-one of the scheduled radiation treatments, he would grant to me a four-week reprieve before beginning the final phase of treatment, yet another chemotherapy drug. I was keeping my eye on that promise.

As painful and difficult as radiation therapy was, I continued to search for bright spots in the darkness. Occasionally, I found one. Immediately following my final radiation treatment, I had a humorous occasion to remind Dr. Stone of the promise of reprieve that he had given to me. I had been prescribed some pain medication that I used sparingly due to the fact that I am, let's just say, a "light weight" when it comes to drugs. For me, it's kind of like Brill Cream, "a little dab will do you." I was hurting. The term "scalded dog" comes to mind. After having taken the usual half of a pain pill but feeling little to no relief, my husband urged me to go ahead and take the other half, something he would later regret. Taking his advice, I swallowed the pill. The pain then began to ease, giving me some relief.

Then Bobby drove me to the cancer center for an appointment to have my port flushed. By the time I had gotten in to see the nurse, the drugs were beginning to take serious effect on me. Alarmed, the nurse went immediately to fetch the doctor. When he walked in, he stood looking at me for only a moment before exclaiming, "She's drunk!" As I sat slumped in my chair giggling, I explained to him that the pain had been unbearable; therefore I had taken the whole pill this time. He laughingly replied, "Well, you don't seem to be in pain anymore." The nurses, who knew me well, were struggling not to laugh out loud. Dr. Stone, utterly amazed at the idea that one pill would put anybody in the state that I was obviously in, inquired of my husband as to how many of the pain pills I had really taken.

My husband honestly replied, "Only one."

Astonished, Dr. Stone responded, "One pill doesn't do this to anyone."

"It does to her," my husband assured him. Dr. Stone then suggested that two Tylenol followed by two Motrin might be more suitable for me given my obvious intolerance to stronger medication. Four more pills! He had to be kidding me. I, so tired of having to swallow pills on what seemed like a continual basis, crossed my eyes at him while sticking out my tongue like a kindergartener not getting her way. I then declared that I was sick of being sick and sick of having to take more pills. He jokingly suggested that perhaps it would be better for me to stop the pain pills, to go home, and have a strong drink instead. He then turned to my husband telling him to bring me back in a couple of weeks.

"A couple of weeks! What do you mean a couple of weeks?" I yelled at him. By this time, the pain medication had taken complete control of me. What happened next will always be something that I wish I could forget. I have a vague recollection of pointing my finger at him, wagging it, as I, in a drug-induced slur, reminded him, "You promised me four weeks." By now, my husband had told me, the nurses were leaving the room to avoid laughing out loud in front of me. Their laughter echoed down the hall as they watched me leaving, amused at my display of out-of-character behavior. Bobby, with his arm around me, quickly escorted me from the building, while whispering in my ear, "Don't look at anyone, don't talk to anyone," in a futile attempt to stop the hemorrhaging of my mouth.

During the drive home, the pain medication began to wear off. Thinking back to the afternoon, I asked Bobby, "Am I going to be embarrassed later when my mind clears up?"

"Oh yeah!"

Never one for letting things go, I continued, "On a scale of one to ten, just how embarrassed should I be?"

"About a twelve," he joked.

This will forever go into my personal book of my most embarrassing moments! Luckily, Dr. Stone gave me the four-week reprieve and held no ill will at my drug-induced outburst.

Just as I was beginning to feel better, the four weeks was over. I couldn't believe how quickly the time had flown by. I felt that I was just getting started with my life again when it was time to return to the cancer center to begin the final element in my treatment regimen. There was one chemotherapy drug that Dr. Stone thought would be beneficial to me, but I could not have this particular drug during my pregnancy. Now that I was no longer pregnant and had finished radiation, it was to time to get started with this last round of chemotherapy.

When the day arrived for me to begin this drug called Oxaliplatin, I felt so discouraged to be facing three more months of chemotherapy. I had already been doing this for almost a year. I had grown so weary from the war I was fighting to feel good. It seemed that just as I was beginning to win the war, I would be bombed with another treatment just to hit the ground, once again losing the battle. I had one more round to go. So, like a good soldier, I dug in my heels, gritted my teeth, and prepared for the beginning of the end of this ordeal.

This treatment started like all the rest. First, to the scales to weigh-in and then to the lab to have blood drawn, a quick visit with the good doctor, and I was off to the treatment room. I took a seat, waiting patiently for my port to be accessed. *Man, I do not want to be here*, I thought to myself. I hated leaving my children on the days that I had treatment, and now I had a new baby at home to consider as well. I was ready to get this show on the road, being that treatments usually took most of the day. I wanted it over with as quickly as possible so that I could get back to my family.

Knowing that I am often especially sensitive to medications, I hoped I would be able to tolerate this new drug that I was about to receive. With my port finally accessed, anti-nausea medication and steroids were the first to be administered. Once these bags had flowed empty, it was time to begin the dreaded Oxaliplatin. Chandler had taken this chemotherapy drug as part of his treatment. He assured me I would get through it, but it would definitely be different than what I had previously experienced. As the Oxaliplatin began to flow into my body, I waited. I didn't feel any different. *Okay*, I thought, *it is going to be okay*. Bobby was with me, and we sat chatting as we waited for the IV bag to empty. It was a pleasant time. With four children, we rarely have uninterrupted time together to just sit and talk. I enjoyed this time alone with him.

As the treatment was about to end, Bobby suggested that we go ahead to the checkout desk as it is often a long process to get checked out and scheduled for the next appointment. That sounded like a good idea to me. I had a speaking engagement that evening, so we were in a bit of a hurry. Pulling my IV cart behind me, we started to walk toward the checkout area. Suddenly, I felt a lump in my throat that made it difficult to swallow. *Strange*, I thought. I remembered that Chandler had mention that cold drinks could make it feel as though my throat was closing up. He had told me that if that were to happen to not panic. Although it might feel like I couldn't breathe, it would be just a feeling. I would be breathing. I considered that the air in the office was quite chilly. Perhaps the cold air was creating the sensation Chandler had warned me about. I mention to Bobby that I felt a little bit funny. He suggested that we walk back to the nurses' station. Good suggestion.

By the time we got there, as I tried to tell the nurse what was wrong, I noticed that I was stuttering. Frustration built up in me. Why couldn't I talk plainly? I noticed Bobby staring at me, shock and fear written clearly on his face. I felt someone push a chair up under me as I unwillingly sat down. By this time, I was shaking all over as though I was having a seizure. I was embarrassed by all the attention that was being drawn to me. Desperately trying to stop my hands from shaking, I sat on them, but it didn't work. I wanted whatever was happening to stop. People were staring. I heard the nurse that was now sitting in a chair across from me yelling something about "stat" as she explained to me that I was having a panic attack. I knew better. I had suffered from panic attacks when I was in college. Believe me, this was no panic attack. I was doing my best to tell her that she was wrong, but all that I could muster was a feeble attempt at talking. I didn't know it at that time, but I was having an allergic reaction to the chemo drug.

Someone had apparently gone to get Dr. Stone as he suddenly appeared beside me. In an apparent attempt to keep me calm, he joked with me, saying, "You'll do anything to get attention." I was hurt. I searched his face for a hint as to his thoughts. He must be teasing, but I couldn't be certain. Surely, he had to know that I would never do this to myself on purpose. I looked again at Bobby, the look on his face telling me that I was in trouble. The nurse continued to push drugs into my IV. These were to stop the effects of the allergic reaction that I was experiencing. Bobby later told me that he had been expecting me to fall over dead. He had thought I was dying, and nothing had ever scared him that badly in all his life.

I spent the next day in the hospital. It was more than a week before I could speak without stuttering. I spent days in the bed. Too weak to get up, I lay there praying for God to make me feel better. I slept, waking up often to find myself soaking wet with sweat. Then the chills would come, causing me to shiver as if with fever although my temperature remained normal. When would this suffering end? I had been through so much already.

Periodically, Bobby would wake me up in an effort to persuade me to eat; I just couldn't. Nothing was appealing. I had no appetite. Still, he would pester me, begging me to at least drink something and threatening to take me back to the hospital if I refused. Believing the only way to get him to leave me alone was to drink, I consented to sipping some hot tea. It would be weeks before I could tolerate anything cold. I was absolutely miserable, laying there feeling sorry for myself.

Still not understanding what had happened to me, I cried, believing that I would have to continue treatment, receiving this same drug that had left me bedridden. Chandler had been right, this was definitely different than my previous experience with chemotherapy. Day turned into night. Another day passed. When would I ever begin to feel better? Having experienced some of these same side effects, Chandler encouraged me by promising that each day I would get a little better. *Little*, apparently, was the key word.

When Dr. Stone called me the next week, he explained to me that I'd had a severe allergic reaction to Oxaliplatin. Had I left the cancer center before the allergic reaction began, the results would have been tragic. Again, God had kept me alive for a purpose. Dr. Stone informed me that I could never have

Oxaliplatin again. With that, my treatment was complete. I barely stifled a scream of excitement. I couldn't believe that he was really telling me it was over. I confirmed that Dr. Stone did believe that the treatment I'd received was sufficient, that nothing was being compromised by my finishing early. As I was hanging up the phone, I walked into my daughter's room and shut the door. I fell to the floor with tears pouring out. It was over, finally over. Today was a new day, a bright day, sunny and crisp. It was a beautiful day, and it was the first day of the rest of my life.

God again used something that seemed and felt terrible at the time to bring good. Although I still faced months of fighting off the lasting effects of the chemotherapy drugs, this time when I felt better, it would last. There would be no more poison flowing through my veins making me sick. No more lost battles. The war had been won. It was finished! I could hardly believe that the ordeal was over. Now was the time for my ministry to begin. God had been preparing me. Now he was calling. It was time to go tell what he had done for me.

Cancer: My Friend

Having cancer has forever changed my life for the good, teaching me many valuable lessons, shaping my perspective to recognize the things that are truly important. Along the way, I learned how to have fun in the midst of despair, not allowing our circumstances to determine my joy. I learned to look for every opportunity to enjoy life even when life didn't make sense. I learned that the things that have to get done will get done. Not that I have ever been a June Cleaver, but order in the house went from bad to worse as clutter took over. The mountain of laundry became a threatening avalanche as more clean clothes were piled on top. I discovered that life as we know it did not end when my children had to dig through that mountain to find something clean to wear. One child would balance the pile while another would carefully extract the desired article. With a hard shake to remove wrinkles, the clothes were then donned and worn.

The children always had something to eat, clothes to wear, and a roof over their heads. Things may not have been exactly as we wanted, but we always had everything we needed. As long as my children know Christ as their Savior and know that I love them, everything else is small stuff. Things that used to drive me crazy just don't seem so important anymore. Time. Time is the most precious resource I have. How I spend it will be my legacy. I ask myself, do I want my children to remember that the bathroom was always clean, or do I want them to remember that Mama had fun playing monopoly with them? Do I want them to remember that the kitchen floor got swept every night, or that Mama took a walk with them while they shared about the day they'd had? The answers to these questions are obvious.

When I began to write about my experience of being pregnant while having cancer, I realized just how deeply affected all the members of my family had been by this experience. I asked each one of the children to sit down and tell me in his or her own words what it had felt like to have a mommy with cancer. Bobby agreed to talk about his thoughts and feelings as well. Here are their stories.

Bobby's Story: In His Words

When Amy asked me to tell what her experience with cancer was like for me, I really didn't know where to start. I didn't realize just how hard writing about her ordeal must have been for her until I started contemplating my experiences and feelings. I guess that I should say our experiences since cancer affects so much more than just the person who is sick. I would describe it as an atomic bomb detonated at the ground level of the family. Its ever-expanding concentric rings of fear and influence ripped throughout the family, the church, friends, and the community at large with the maximum devastation occurring at the nucleus of the family. And just like Hiroshima and Nagasaki, it comes without warning. Unsuspected and unprepared for, it lands with full force. That is how I would describe the influence of cancer on any given family. But it wasn't any given family! It was *my* family! When you see the mushroom cloud rising in the distance on the horizon and those concentric rings arrive at your doorstep in the form of news about a coworker or a neighbor down the road or a friend of a friend, you say, "That's bad," or "I am really sorry to hear that." You may try to reach out by carrying them a meal or sending a card, but ultimately it is someone else's family, someone else's issue. But when the A-bomb—or maybe I should say the C-bomb—lands on *your* house, you find yourself in a very different situation.

Amy is a wonderful wife. God knew what he was doing when he placed us together. Our personalities complement each other perfectly. She is the best mother any child could ever wish for, always placing the needs of the children ahead of her own. Professionally, I am a civil engineer, a logical thinker, a problem solver. Personally, I am an avid outdoorsman, part-time farmer, your quintessential country boy—a survivor. I built the house we live in. We grow and can a portion of our own food. Each year, we strive to become more self-sufficient. These qualities in me bring comfort to Amy in a world that does not seem to be changing for the better. Amy and I have a lot of things in common: a love for rural country living, desire for self-reliance, and wanting to raise our children in a God-fearing home, but we are polar opposites in some respects. Such is the case when it comes to our personalities. Amy tends to be more high strung, and I am more laid-back (most of the time) except for when she, under the influence of chemotherapy, gets a wild idea to operate the tractor and bushhog, destroying some of my tools in the process. I guess you might say that in some situations, my personality has a calming effect on her.

When Amy began having symptoms, we went to the doctor. We were awaiting the results from the testing that was done. In true fashion, Amy was somewhat apprehensive, and I was a little more relaxed, not wanting to borrow trouble. Amy called me at work and was scared as she informed me that the doctor's office had called and told her to be in the office at 9:00 a.m. the following morning and to bring her husband. Now I was scared! I knew this could not be good. This kind of urgency is not common for a doctor's office. The next morning, we learned that my wife had colon cancer.

Years ago, our first child was delivered by emergency C-section. I was allowed in the operating room to observe although I am not sure why. Every time Amy had a contraction, Jonathan's (our son) heart rate would drop. I don't know if the umbilical cord was somehow restricted, but it was not your quintessential C-section. (I have observed three more since that time.) I have seen less blood at a hog killing. I don't blink an eye at gutting a deer, but that was my wife's intestines on the OR table. I was terrified, and she looked at me from the table as if requesting loving reassurance. I put on my best poker face and determined in my mind that I would not let her see my fear.

Once again, as we received the news about my wife's cancer, I put on my best game face and tried to be that calm, relaxed, comforting husband that my wife needed. Besides, all we knew was that she had cancer, we did not know if it had spread or in what stage the cancer might exist. I had to think in these terms because that was the only way (as I perceived) that I could find hope in spite of the words the doctor had just spoken to us. What I felt is hard to explain. It was as if I went into survival mode. I was nauseated, but at the same time, it felt like an adrenalin rush. My mind went numb. It was as if the psychological portion of my brain understood the danger and level of stress I was to come under and took over. It would limit what I could think about. It would not allow me to delve completely into the situation in which I found myself. Besides, I had to be strong for Amy. Then there was the next consideration, Amy was pregnant.

The doctor scheduled the operation and recommended the best surgeon that she knew, but how would the surgery affect the new life growing in my wife's womb? She had suffered a miscarriage several weeks earlier, and I could hardly bear the thought of her having to repeat the physical and mental anguish she endured. The problems that existed in my life up until that time seemed to fade into oblivion. The worst economy since the Great Depression, a highly political and stressful job, and projects left incomplete at home were no longer important. I stayed in this condition until the time for the surgery. I prayed many times for my wife's health, especially prior to going into surgery. During surgery, I was scared and nervous, but once again, my mind would not allow contemplation of the what ifs. Friends and family waited with me during the surgery, trying their best to comfort me, but the effect was little more than an attempted distraction. Some relief came when the nurse informed me that Amy's operation was over and it had gone well. Greater relief came when the surgeon came out and informed me that he thought he had removed all the cancer. Now I could breathe a little bit; we simply had to get Amy recovered from the surgery.

Her first night was horrible. She was so sick! The pain medication was making her throw up, and she said the room was spinning. She intentionally took herself off the pain medication until the nausea improved. Friends and family did their best to support me during this time. I will always be grateful for the prayers and support, but deep down inside, I felt alone, as if I was the only one going through this ordeal. During the next couple of days, Amy began to improve, and I started feeling better. The relief did not last however; the gastroenterologist that had found Amy's cancer came and told us that the biopsy taken during surgery had been processed. She told us that the cancer had spread into a lymph node. The surgery had apparently not been as successful as we had hoped it would be. With the spread into the lymph node, her situation was much more grave.

As strong as I thought I was emotionally and as much as I knew that Amy needed me to be strong, I could no longer hold back the tears flowing from my eyes. I am not sure if Amy had ever seen me cry. Even though I was crying, I was still trying to hold myself together. A short while later when I could excuse myself, I left the room for a few minutes and broke down completely, crying as hard as I ever have in my life. My mental self-defense mechanism that I had been leaning on since we learned that Amy had cancer, was no longer relevant. I had been forced to contemplate things I did not want to face, and on top of everything I was trying to deal with, my wife was pregnant.

An oncologist was assigned to Amy, and in his initial visit, he explained to us about the various stages of cancer and what they meant. He spoke in terms of statistics that I understood all too well but was not sure Amy fully comprehended in her drug-induced state. He initially gave her a 45 percent chance of survival. I sank to depths that I have never known. I was terrified. We had three children at that time that needed their mama. The thought of those kids growing up without their mother was horrible. The thought of me trying to raise them by myself terrified me. How could I honor my wife's wishes and home-school our children (as she had been doing) and earn a living at the same time? All the thousands of things that she does for those kids each day—that I know I could never do as well, if at all. How could I do without my wife who lovingly supports me in so many ways? I may support her financially, but she supports me in ways that money cannot buy. She is truly the keystone to our family. Then the question came: why? I got a sick feeling in the depth of my gut.

I have grown exponentially in the Lord during the time of and after the predicament, but at that point, I would not say I was where I should be in my Christian journey. For years I had felt the Lord calling me to do something, but I had not been obedient. I kept putting him off and not reconciling the situation with the Lord. Now I had an overwhelming sense that the cancer my wife had was the Lord's judgment on me for being disobedient. I felt as though the weight of the world was on my shoulders. My dear precious wife was suffering, and it was my fault. I could hardly bear the thought of all the pain and grief I would be causing. I felt like the scum of the earth. My talents and abilities and the securities my wife took in them were useless in this situation. This was one problem the engineer could not solve and the country boy could not fix. To make it worse, I was the cause.

I prayed often but felt as if God was not listening because of my disobedience. I'm not really sure how I survived and functioned during this time. I guess the Lord carried me. The gastroenterologist, surgeon, and the ob-gyn began telling Amy that she must abort if she wanted to live. This only made my problem worse. Would I now be responsible for two deaths? Words cannot describe the torment to which I was exposed.

My wife, being the wonderful Christian woman that she is, took a stand. She was several days out from the surgery now, and with some of the drugs wearing off, she was in more of her normal mind-set. She told the doctor she would not have an abortion. The stand she took, the strength she displayed, and her assurance that she's doing the right thing (as she understood it) unto the Lord encouraged and strengthened me. She said, as she lay in the hospital room, "The Lord knew I had cancer before I got pregnant." We may not have known it at that time, but this was a turning point. The Lord was calling Amy to trust in him. During the next several weeks, she came to a point of surrender to his will, whatever that will would be. Almost immediately, God gave us hope for Amy's survival when she saw the oncologist to schedule chemotherapy. Yet I still heard a calling from God for my own surrender and obedience. When I prayed for my wife or anything else, it was as if God was telling me, "Do what I told you to do, and I will answer your prayers." Finally, sufficiently broken, I surrendered to the Lord's will and immediately felt years of burden lifted from me. The Holy Spirit strengthened me, and prayers that had remained unanswered for years became reality. Now I felt that the prayers for my wife would be truly heard by God. Amy completed her chemotherapy, gave birth to Joshua, and then underwent radiation.

All in all, it was a tremendous valley we had to cross, but when I look back, I can see how God used our situation for his glory in many different ways. My wife has an unbelievable testimony, and I got my life right with the Lord. The lessons that I learned from the entire ordeal was something I heard before but had never resonated with me completely until I was placed in this situation. I learned that God is faithful. He always does what he says he will do. Also I learned that there is no safer place to be than slapdab in the middle of God's will. Because when you are in his will, regardless of what happens, you are a winner. The situation will either resolve itself to your good (as it did in our situation) or God will take you on to paradise. You're a winner either way.

The urging of the Lord that Amy and I felt on our lives comes because we are Christians. You must first be saved and have a relationship with God through Christ Jesus before you can understand the Lord's calling in your life. Once saved, the Holy Spirit will indwell with you, and through reading God's Word, he will lead you in the paths you should take. If you are not saved, I encourage you to ask the Lord Jesus into your heart. You must acknowledge that you are a sinner and understand that sin is punishable by death. You must also understand that Jesus, who is God's son, died on the cross for your sins. You must repent of your sins and ask the Lord Jesus to forgive your sins (he is the only one who can) and ask him to come into your heart and live in you.

Jonathan's Story

I was very worried that my mom was going to die. I was worried because when I saw people coming up to my mom crying, I didn't understand because she told me everything would be fine. The toughest part was going so long without seeing my mom. She was in the hospital for a long time. Dad didn't come home either. I was without both of my parents for ten days. On day seven, I saw a gray truck coming down the road. I thought that it looked like my dad's truck, but it couldn't possibly be him. It started to turn in. It was my dad! I couldn't believe it was really him! Luke and I ran to greet him. He took us to the hospital to see Mom for the first time. Mom was drugged. When we had to leave, we really didn't want to go. Luke and Emma cried. When Mom finally came home, she looked like she just had gotten out of bed. A lot of people came to help us out while Mom was sick. It was like a feast, there was so much food. It was Luke's birthday when she came home. When Mom stepped out of the truck, she was holding a party balloon. The next day, we played baseball for Luke's birthday party.

We had to get used to Mama being in the bathroom all the time. She was very sick. Luke, Emma, Dad, and I had to use the bathroom outside sometimes. My grandmother stayed with us for a long time. I was mad at her because I wanted my mom to take care of me, not her. I'm not mad at her anymore. My mom couldn't do much because she was so sick. I was upset that I had to stop taking karate lessons. I helped my mom take care of Luke and Emma sometimes. My friend Lex's mom came over a lot to help. I liked when they came over because I got to play with my friend Lex and his brother Logan.

I was worried about my mom losing the baby. I remember when the other babies died. It was a really sad time. I was scared that something would be wrong with the baby because of the chemotherapy. Radiation treatments were really hard for my mom. I was really glad when my mom started to feel better. I feel like we are finally coming out of the darkness.

Luke's Story

When I went to see my mom at the hospital, she played UNO with us. I was sad because my mom was in the hospital. When she came home, she brought us a heart for Valentine's Day. We had a baseball birthday party for me. My aunt made me a baseball cake. My grandmother was at our house a whole lot. It was easy to trick her into letting me stay up late playing with my toys. I was very glad when Mama came home. I missed my mom when she was gone.

Emma's Story

I cried a lot when Mama was sick. I did not like it when I had to leave her at the hospital. We took her a valentine card to the hospital. She asked the doctor for some tape to hang our cards up on the wall. I thought it was funny to ask a doctor for tape. When my mom needed the nurse, she let me push the button to make the nurse come to her room.

When my mom came home, there were lots of people coming to our house. The doctor told Mama that she wasn't supposed to hold us, but she did it anyway. I really liked it when daddy played Candy Land with me. I didn't like Mama being pregnant. She looked mean and scary when she was sick. She wasn't really mean. My mama is nice.

Joshua's Story

For you created my inmost being;
You knit me together in my mother's womb.
I praise you because I am fearfully and wonder-
fully made;
Your works are wonderful, I know that full well.

Psalms 139:13–14 (NIV)

Conclusion

A visiting pastor at our church once stated, "Those whom God uses mightily suffer mightily." That quote really resonated with me. As I began to reflect on the lives of some of the greatest men in the Bible, I recognized the truth of that statement. Joseph was sold into slavery by his own brothers. Paul was jailed unjustly. God allowed Satan to test Job by taking all his worldly possessions, including his family. These men are only a few of the mighty warriors of the Bible who suffered for the kingdom of God. I have come to recognize that it is a privilege to be found worthy by God to be used for his glory.

As more people hear our story, we are encouraged to know that God has used us to reach out and inspire others. The interest in our experience has often taken me very much by surprise. The more we go to churches to tell our story, the more we are asked to go. Yet my story does not seem like a big deal to me. It wasn't a story to me, it was simply my life. We are just ordinary people whom God chose for this purpose.

This past year has forever changed my life for the good. By traveling through many deep valleys and cresting many tall mountains, I have grown closer to God, learning to trust his will no matter how frightening it may seem. God has given me a new appreciation for the many blessings that I used to take for granted. I have learned to live without fear, knowing that God is in control. I have learned to find joy and purpose in each day. Every day that I wake up is a good day.

As Joshua is approaching a year old, I sit in awe at the journey that we have taken. He is a healthy baby boy reaching all the age-appropriate milestones. People still stare at him in wonder as they exclaim to me, "Well, he looks so normal." That is because he is normal. God used Joshua and me to show his power. God is faithful. He has proven to me that he can be trusted in all things. I enjoy just sitting in the living room floor watching the beautiful little miracle that God gave to me while he plays. The tears come anew every time I consider that if I had been a different person in a different place with different experiences, I may have killed my baby. Thank God that he gave me enough mercy and grace to trust him. I have lived a miracle and can testify to the goodness of our God.

Today, as I praise God that I am cancer-free, I am getting back to the task of living. I have lessons to teach, gardens to plant, bread to bake, dishes to wash, diapers to change, the never ending "Mom, I'm hungry," to pay attention to, and a mountain of laundry to wash. I love my life! I will never take my blessings for granted again! Every day I thank God for letting me be his vessel, Bobby's wife, and my children's mother.

In obedience to God's calling, we are available to share our story with anyone or any organization. The Bible tells us that we were created to bring glory to God. It is my honor and my privilege to have suffered that others may see the power of our God.

Afterword

If you are fifty years old or older or if you have a family history of colon cancer, please get a colonoscopy! No, it is not fun, but it is like a day at the beach compared to chemotherapy and radiation. Just do it. It could save your life. It saved mine.

Pregnancy combined with cancer is a terrible place to land, but it is not hopeless! In the medical field, there remains yet much ignorance as to treatment options for pregnant women. The field is changing as research is now supporting the possibility of having chemotherapy while pregnant with positive results. Always get a second opinion or third or fourth, but never give up.

Finally, God is always in control. His will is perfect even when we don't understand it. God is faithful and can always be trusted.

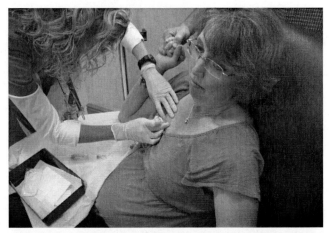

Amy getting chemotherapy during her pregnancy.

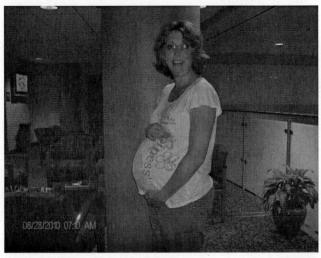

August 28, 2010 just moments before we got to meet our Joshua.

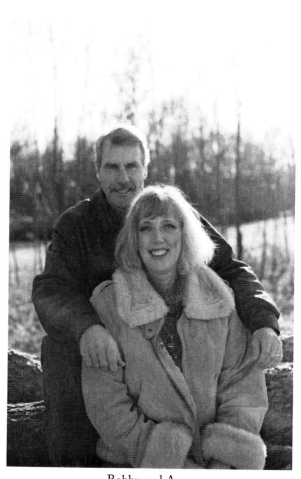

Bobby and Amy

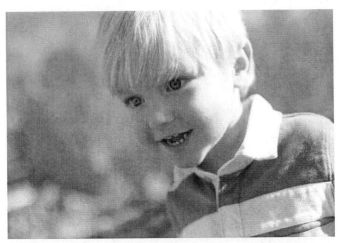

Joshua Hodges Hanley at two years old.

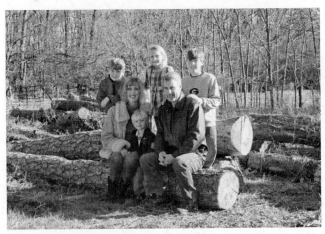

The Hanley family in December 2012. Amy,
Joshua, Bobby, Luke, Emma, and Jonathan.

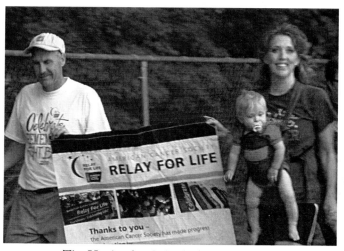

The Hanley family leading the Survivor's
lap at Relay for Life 2011.